Brian V. Reamy

Editor

Hyperlipidemia Management for Primary Care

An Evidence-Based Approach

Foreword by Charles E. Henley

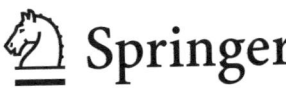 Springer

Editor

Brian V. Reamy, MD
Uniformed Services University of the Health Sciences
Bethesda, MD
USA

ISBN: 978-0-387-76605-8   e-ISBN: 978-0-387-76606-5
DOI: 10.1007/978-0-387-76606-5

Library of Congress Control Number: 2008924799

Printed on acid-free paper

9 8 7 6 5 4 3 2 1

springer.com

To my patients: You have taught me so much over the years.
To my friends: Your humor and companionship keep me smiling and balanced.
To my wife and daughter, Dianne and Katie: your constant support and love keep me whole.

Hyperlipidemia Management for Primary Care

Foreword

One of the possible benefits of 30 years of medical practice is the ability to develop some sense of perspective with regard to major transitions in medicine. Many physicians who graduated from medical school in the mid- to late 1970s may recall feeling less than comfortable about counseling patients regarding lifestyle modification and heart disease risk. A total cholesterol of 250 mg% at that time was considered within normal limits. The best information on the causation of heart disease came from epidemiologic data showing associations between increased consumption of dairy products and fat in the industrialized countries of northern Europe and America, and a corresponding increase in morbidity and mortality from heart disease as compared to other countries that were less well developed or as compared to Mediterranean countries, where there was a different type of diet lower in saturated fats and cholesterol.

Treatment options in those days were based more on anecdotal information and observation than on evidence. The idea that coronary artery disease was an inflammatory problem in which the main culprit was oxidized LDL and the idea that heart disease risk could be managed had not yet made the transition to clinical practice. This attitude all changed as information from the largest and longest running prospective epidemiologic study on heart disease—the Framingham Study—began publishing data on causality and risk factors. Although it takes time for information to find its way into clinical practice, the evidence produced from the Framingham Study was powerful and influenced clinical practice in profound ways. We now had good clinical evidence for causation and the contribution of total cholesterol, LDL, and other major risk factors such as diabetes, obesity, and hypertension. More than that, we could now identify a risk category for our patients. Coupled with the Framingham Study were the National Cholesterol Education Program (NCEP) and the Adult Treatment Panel (ATP) I, II, and III. In fact, one can follow the progression of our knowledge of the effect of drug therapy with statins by following the NCEP/ATP trials, which developed the original framework for management of LDL in patients with CHD and demonstrated the effect of even more rigorous management of LDL, even to the point of reversal of plaque.

These clinical milestones and the case for why we should care about data from drug trials have been carefully laid out and validated in this new book edited by Dr. Brian Reamy, using the results from the clinical trials themselves. From the large primary prevention trials to the newer trials such as PROVE-IT-TIMI and the REVERSAL trial, we can see why and how the evidence for LDL management has been translated into practice, with a reduction in risk for heart disease. Many of these trials have been essential to our understanding of the effect of HMG-CoA reductase in lowering LDL and raising HDL. The authors are gifted in the way they use information from the literature to anticipate the questions we would ask ourselves as practitioners about the role of the statins in reducing cardiovascular risk.

We now find ourselves in the midst of an explosion of information on cholesterol and lipids. At times, this can be intimidating to the clinician trying to understand the significance of the data on pathophysiology and treatment options with respect to a patient with a particular risk profile. What has been needed is a comprehensive, evidence-based assessment of our understanding of the relationships effecting cardiovascular disease and the various interventions and treatment options available. But, more than that, we need to know what works.

This book treats physicians intelligently by providing a deeper understanding of why we know what we know and how this information fits into a holistic view of overall patient care, not just how it fits into cutoff levels for various laboratory results. It is written from the perspective of a family physician with many years of clinical experience and seasoning in academic medicine. Chapter 10 contains eight cases that illustrate how the evidence from clinical trials and the information from the book can be used to treat patients. This book should be well received by anyone seeking to understand the complex realm of hyperlipidemia and hypercholesterolemia more completely.

Dr. Brian Reamy, the editor and principal author of this work, is a nationally recognized educator with a profound respect for the doctor–patient relationship and for the need for physicians to use evidence for the benefit of their patients. He and his contributors have created a seminal work by virtue of its comprehensiveness and its validation of the literature. This book will certainly find its place as a resource for physicians in the war against preventable heart disease.

Charles E. Henley, DO, MPH,
Colonel MC, USA (Retired)
Professor and Vice Chair
Department of Family Medicine
Founders and Associates Research Chair
in Family Medicine
University of Oklahoma College
of Medicine–Tulsa
Tulsa, OK
USA

Preface

Cardiovascular disease remains the leading killer of Americans. Since 2003, it has also become the leading cause of death of in other parts of the world. As public sanitation and the eradication of common infectious illnesses have progressed, cardiovascular disease has risen in prevalence worldwide. Several studies have shown that the four conventional risk factors of smoking, diabetes, hypertension, and hyperlipidemia are present in more than 80% to 90% of patients with coronary heart disease (CHD). Other studies have also shown that optimal care for hyperlipidemia is provided to only 18% to 48% of patients with this problem, despite the fact that most patients' cardiovascular risk can be dramatically reduced with lifestyle changes or with the addition of a single medication.

The reasons for this poor implementation are many. They range from inadequate or outdated information to poor compliance by our patients as a consequence of misplaced fears or incorrect knowledge of dietary and lifestyle interventions. System problems with the identification of patients with hyperlipidemia and the ongoing delivery of optimal care are significant and necessitate excellent patient education and empowerment. Each patient should have an individualized and well-understood "prescription" for prevention of cardiovascular disease that incorporates diet, physical activity, and, in some cases, medication. By empowering our patients to control their hyperlipidemia, we can help reduce the burden of this prevalent disease.

Indeed, the optimum control of hyperlipidemia provides primary care physicians with an extraordinary opportunity to prevent cardiovascular disease in their patients. Both *primary prevention* (prevention of CHD before any clinical manifestations) and *secondary prevention* (prevention of recurrent CHD after an initial clinical event) are possible. In fact, powerful new evidence supports the concept that reducing low density lipoprotein cholesterol (LDL-C) to levels below 70 mg/dl may lead to remodeling and the reversal of existing atherosclerosis.

This volume addresses the extensive evidence base that already exists to support the treatment of hyperlipidemia. It reviews current national guidelines and provides extensive information on lifestyle changes and nondrug treatment for hyperlipidemia. Our patients have many appropriate questions about highly publicized diets and therapeutic foods. This book provides the primary physician with the best evidence-based information available to help address common questions about diets, foods, herbs, and supplements. Drug treatment, drug interactions, and drugs in development are discussed, and an evidence-based approach to their utilization is offered.

Practicing clinicians are also confronted with special populations such as the elderly, women, or elite athletes who present special treatment challenges that are addressed in this book. Important issues regarding novel screening methods are reviewed, and a practical approach to the patient with hyperlipidemia is outlined. The penultimate section of the book provides a case-based discussion of some of the difficult, but fairly common, situations confronted by most primary care clinicians and offers an approach to each. Anticipated future directions in the treatment of hyperlipidemia are discussed in the final chapter.

The past 20 years have seen extraordinary advances in the treatment of CHD. The rapid rise in the incidence of this disease has been slowed. New medications, invasive vascular techniques, enhanced strategies, and protocols to govern treatment in the acute ischemic setting have all progressed substantially. HMG-CoA reductase inhibitor medications (statins) have become a standard part of treatment in acute coronary syndromes.

Against this background of success in acute interventions, the evidence regarding the etiology and prevention of cardiovascular disease has also grown substantially. It is time that optimum prevention of cardiovascular disease helps to reduce the burden of this horrible illness. The tools and methods are available to all physicians: It is time to employ them.

This book represents the cumulative wisdom of years in practice of a group of physicians who believe that prevention of cardiovascular disease through the control of hyperlipidemia is an achievable and extremely important goal. It is a goal that motivated us to write this book and will, we hope, inspire readers to optimize the treatment of hyperlipidemia for each of their patients.

Brian V. Reamy, MD
Colonel, USAF, MC

Contents

Contributors

Erika V. Barger, MD, LtCol, USAF, MC
Chief, Medical Staff, 579th Medical Group, Bolling Air Force Base,
Washington, DC

James W. Haynes, MD, LtCol, USAF, MC
Program Director, Headquarters Air Armament Center Family Medicine Residency,
Department of Family Medicine, Eglin Air Force Base Hospital, FL

Allyson S. Howe, MD, CAQ Sports Medicine, Maj, USAF, MC
Residency Teaching Staff Physician, Director of Sports Medicine, Department of
Family Medicine, Malcolm Grow Medical Center, Andrews Air Force Base, MD

Christopher G. Jarvis, MD, Maj, MC, USA
Director, Sports Medicine, Department of Primary Care, Blanchfield Army
Community Hospital, LaPointe Health Clinic, Fort Campbell, KY

Sarah Sallee Jones, MD, Maj, USAF, MC
Associate Program Director, Family Medicine Residency, Department of Family
Medicine, David Grant Medical Center, Travis Air Force Base, CA

Brian V. Reamy, MD, Col, USAF, MC
Chair and Associate Professor, Department of Family Medicine, Uniformed
Services University of the Health Sciences, Bethesda, MD
breamy@usuhs.mil

Brian K. Unwin, MD, Col, MC, USA
Vice-Chair and Assistant Professor, Department of Family Medicine, Uniformed
Services University of the Health Sciences, Bethesda, MD

Christopher W. Walker, MD, Maj, USAF, MC
Associate Program Director, David Grant Family Medicine Residency Program,
Department of Family Medicine, University of California at Davis Affiliate
Program/David Grant Medical Center, Travis Air Force Base, CA

Chapter 1
Overview of Evidence Supporting the Treatment of Hyperlipidemia

Brian V. Reamy

Introduction

Multiple basic science studies have established that atherosclerosis is much more than the mere accumulation of excess lipid in the walls of arteries leading to progressive narrowing of the vessel. Instead, it should be thought of as an inflammatory disease involving many cellular and molecular responses. Inflammatory cells and mediators participate at every stage of atherogenesis, from the earliest fatty streak to the most advanced fibrous lesion [1]. Elevated glucose, increased blood pressure, and inhaled cigarette by-products can trigger and perpetuate inflammation. However, one of the key factors triggering this inflammation is oxidized LDL (low density lipoprotein). When excess LDL is taken up by macrophages, it triggers the release of inflammatory mediators that can lead to thickening and/or rupture of plaque lining the arterial walls. Ruptured or unstable plaques are responsible for clinical events such as myocardial infarction and stroke. Lipid lowering, whether by diet or medication, can therefore be thought of as an *antiinflammatory and plaque-stabilizing therapy* [2].

At What Age Does Atherosclerosis Start?

The emergence of the inflammatory theory of atherogenesis has added interest to the question: At what age does atherosclerosis begin? Evidence from pathological studies has shown that fatty streaks start as early as 2 years of age. In addition, the amount of atherosclerosis present in children and adolescents at autopsy correlates significantly with the key established risk factors of LDL cholesterol, blood pressure, body mass index (BMI), smoking history, and family history [3]. Three key

B.V. Reamy
Chair and Associate Professor, Department of Family Medicine, Uniformed Services University of the Health Sciences, Bethesda, MD
e-mail: breamy@usuhs.mil

B.V. Reamy (ed.), *Hyperlipidemia Management for Primary Care*,
DOI: 10.1007/978-0-387-76606-5_1, © Springer Science+Business Media, LLC 2008

1

long-term studies provide the evidence that atherosclerosis is a largely predictable process that begins in childhood and progresses at a rate determined by coronary risk factors. It is accelerated or decelerated by the accumulation or reduction of those risk factors [4–6]. These three studies are the Pathobiologic Determinants of Atherosclerosis in Youth (PDAY), the Bogalusa Heart Study, and the Muscatine Study [4–6].

Coronary artery risk factors in children and adolescents are associated with the early development of atherosclerosis in adults: these factors include low HDL (high density lipoprotein), high body mass index (BMI), high blood pressure, and high LDL. Startlingly, the carotid intima medial thickness (IMT) of *adults* (a surrogate for systemic atherosclerosis) can be predicted by *childhood* measures of LDL and BMI [7].

Trials focused on the treatment of the young are sparse for reasons of concerns about research in this vulnerable group. However, evidence is slowly accumulating that treatment is feasible and safe in children as young as 8 years of age. Trials have demonstrated the effectiveness of dietary intervention, smoking cessation, exercise, and medications on the reduction of risk factors in the young [8–12]. Whether this early intervention will lead to reduced cardiovascular outcomes later in life has still not been proven.

Pre-Statin Trials

Older trials, done in the 1980s before the advent of statin drugs, provided several insights into the benefits of cholesterol reduction that formed the basis of early practice guidelines from the National Cholesterol Education Program (NCEP). The Lipid Research Clinics Coronary Primary Prevention Cholestyramine Trial showed that lowering cholesterol by 9% resulted in a 19% reduction in coronary heart disease (CHD) morbidity and mortality [13]. The resin agent colestipol was tested in combination with nicotinic acid in the Cholesterol Lowering Atherosclerosis Study (CLAS), and this showed a significant reduction in angiographic progression of atherosclerosis versus a control group receiving no medication [14].

Fibrate agents were also tested in a number of early trials with conflicting results. The Helsinki Heart Study, which tested gemfibrozil, showed reduced CHD mortality but not all-cause mortality [15]. Troublesome results of trials of another fibrate agent, clofibrate, also showed that its use lowered CHD mortality but also led to an unexpected increase in all-cause mortality from violent death. This finding initially tempered enthusiasm for the use of cholesterol-lowering agents [16].

Statin Trials

Against this backdrop of the positive effects of cholesterol lowering on CHD morbidity and mortality and the questionable effects of cholesterol lowering on all-cause mortality, the inhibitors of 3-hydroxy-3-methylglutaryl-coenzyme-A reductase (HMG-CoA reductase) were introduced. These agents inhibit the enzyme that catalyzes the conversion of HMG-CoA to mevalonate; this is an early and rate-limiting step in the biosynthesis of cholesterol. As each of these medications was introduced, its generic name had the suffix *statin*. Subsequently, this entire class of medications has been referred to by the nickname of statins.

These new medications provided much more potency and fewer side effects than the resins, nicotinic acid, and the fibrates that preceded them. However, it took several large prospective, randomized, double-blind trials in the 1990s to move statins from newly introduced to their current status as the workhorses of lipid control. These trials studied the use of statins both for *primary prevention*—treatment of hyperlipidemia in patients without manifest disease—as well as for *secondary prevention*—treatment of hyperlipidemia when clinical disease is already present to prevent recurrent events.

Primary Prevention Statin Trials of the 1990s

The two most significant randomized, controlled, primary prevention trials of the 1990s were the West of Scotland Coronary Prevention Study (WOSCOPS – 1995) and the United States Air Force and University of Texas Coronary Atherosclerosis Prevention Study (AFCAPS/TEXCAPS – 1998) [17,18]. WOSCOPS treated 6596 men with markedly elevated cholesterol levels but no manifest vascular disease with 40 mg/day pravastatin. After just 5 years, coronary events were reduced by 31%, coronary artery disease (CAD) deaths were reduced by 28%, coronary revascularizations were reduced by 37%, and all-cause mortality was reduced by 22%.

The second primary prevention trial was the United States Air Force and University of Texas Coronary Atherosclerosis Prevention Study [18]. This trial treated 6605 patients (15% were women) whose cholesterol values were in the *average range* for the United States population. All were treated with either 20 or 40 mg per day lovastatin. Remarkably, even in this *low-risk* group of patients, after 5 years of therapy, there was a 25% risk reduction in nonfatal myocardial infarction and coronary deaths, a 40% risk reduction in fatal and nonfatal myocardial infarctions, and a 33% reduction in the need for revascularizations (Table 1.1).

Secondary Prevention Statin Trials of the 1990s

Three remaining trials established the use of statins in secondary prevention. The Scandanavian Simvastatin Survival Study (4S – 1994) studied 4444 patients (19% were women) for 5.4 years [19]. Treated patients received either 20 or 40 mg simvastatin per day. The patients were high risk in terms of both the presence of preexisting disease and markedly unfavorable cholesterol profiles. In this study, CAD deaths were reduced by 34%, myocardial infarcts were reduced by 42%, revascularizations were reduced by 37%, and all-cause mortality was reduced by 30%.

The next large study was the Long Term Intervention with Pravastatin in Ischemic Disease Study Group (LIPID – 1998) [20]. This trial followed 9014 patients with

Table 1.1 Major primary prevention trials of statin treatment for coronary heart disease (CHD)

	Number of patients	Men/women (%)	R	Baseline labs (mg/dl)	Posttreatment	Risk reduction (%)
WOSCOPS:	6596	100/0	Pravastatin 40 mg/day	TC = 272	−20%	Nonfatal MI/CHD death, −31%
				LDL = 192	−26%	CHD mortality, −28%
				HDL = 44	+5%	Total mortality, −22%
				TG = 164	−12%	Revascularizations, −37%
AFCAPS/ TEXCAPS:	6605	85/15	Lovastatin 20–40 mg/day	TC = 221	−19%	Nonfatal MI/CHD death, −25%
				LDL = 150	−26%	Fatal/nonfatal MI, −40%
				HDL = 37	+5%	Total mortality, no change
				TG = 158	−13%	Revascularizations, −33%

WOSCOPS, West of Scotland Coronary Prevention Study; 4S, Scandanavian Simvastatin Survival Study; LIPID, Long Term Intervention with Pravastatin Trial; AFCAPS/TEXCAPS, Air Force/Texas Atherosclerosis Prevention Study; CARE, Cholesterol and Recurrent Events; TC, total cholesterol; HDL, high density lipoprotein; TG, triglycerides; LDL, low density lipoprotein; MI, myocardial infarction; CHD, coronary heart disease.

clinical CHD (17% were women) for 6.1 years. All were treated with pravastatin, 40 mg per day. Initial lipid values were similar to U.S. population means. A marked reduction in relative risk for nonfatal infarct, fatal infarct, total mortality, and CHD mortality was observed.

The third major secondary prevention trial was the Cholesterol and Recurrent Events Trial (CARE – 1996) [21]. This study enrolled 4159 patients (14% were women). Interestingly, the cholesterol values of this group were already close to ideal. All were placed on pravastatin, 40 mg per day. Remarkably, nonfatal infarction was reduced by 24%, fatal infarction was reduced by 29%, total mortality was reduced by 22%, and CHD mortality was reduced by 20%. The secondary prevention trials are summarized in Table 1.2. A conceptual summary of these five large primary and secondary prevention trials is presented in Table 1.3.

Major Trials Since 1999

Low HDL

Fibrates were retested in a 1999 Veterans Administration Study (VA-HIT) that evaluated secondary prevention of CHD events in men with a near-normal LDL (mean, 111 mg/dl), but with a suboptimal HDL (less than 40 mg/dl) [22]. Gemfibrozil was used as the trial medication. Of note, despite the initial low LDL levels, there was a 22% reduction in CHD events in just 5 years of use. This finding confirmed the importance of low HDL as a treatment target in addition to elevated LDL and the usefulness of gemfibrozil in reducing clinical outcomes.

Trials Studying Treatment During Acute Ischemia

As data accumulated on statins, it became clear that they had benefits beyond those predicted simply by reduction in serum LDL cholesterol. Chief among these benefits was an antiinflammatory effect. The pleiotropic antiinflammatory effect of statins led to the hypothesis that their use during the acute inflammation of an ischemic event could provide some benefits. Several trials investigated this idea, but the sentinel trial was the 2001 MIRACL Study [23]. This trial studied the effect of 80 mg atorvastatin initiated within 96 h of an acute coronary syndrome. This randomized, double-blind trial enrolled 3086 adults and demonstrated a relative risk reduction of recurrent ischemic events and rehospitalization. There was no significant reduction in the risk of death or cardiac arrest between the placebo and the atorvastatin group [23]. These results and other trial results have led to the commonplace practice of early initiation of statin therapy in the setting of acute ischemia.

Trials Studying Intensive Reduction of LDL Cholesterol

One of the cardinal questions raised by the trials showing the great benefits of lipid lowering in the 1990s was this: At what LDL level would the benefits of statin

Table 1.2 Major secondary prevention trials of statin treatment for coronary heart disease (CHD)

	Number of patients	Men/women (%)	R	Baseline labs (mg/dl)	Posttreatment	Risk reduction (%)
4S:	4444	81/19	Simvastatin 20–40 mg/day	TC = 261 LDL = 188 HDL = 46 TG = 134	−26% −36% +7% −17%	Nonfatal MI/CHD death, −34% Fatal/nonfatal MI, −42% Total mortality, −30% CHD mortality, −42%
LIPID:	9,014	83/17	Pravastatin 40 mg/day	TC = 218 LDL = 150 HDL = 36 TG = 138	−18% −25% +5% −11%	Nonfatal MI/CHD death, −24% Fatal/nonfatal MI, −29% Total mortality, −22% CHD mortality, −24%
CARE:	4,159	86/14	Pravastatin 40 mg/day	TC = 209 LDL = 139 HDL = 39 TG = 155	−20% −28% +5% −14%	Nonfatal MI/CHD death, −24% Fatal/nonfatal MI, −29% Total mortality, −22% CHD mortality, −20%

WOSCOPS, West of Scotland Coronary Prevention Study; 4S, Scandanavian Simvastatin Survival Study; LIPID, Long Term Intervention with Pravastatin Trial; AFCAPS/TEXCAPS, Air Force/Texas Atherosclerosis Prevention Study; CARE, Cholesterol and Recurrent Events.

Table 1.3 Conceptual model of major statin trials of the 1990s

LDL level (mg/dl) at trial initiation	Patients without CHD: primary prevention	Patients with CHD: secondary prevention
200		
190	WOSCOPS	4S
180		
170		
160		
150	AFCAPS/TEXCAPS	LIPID
140		CARE
130		
120		
110		
100		
	Primary prevention	**Secondary prevention**

WOSCOPS, West of Scotland Coronary Prevention Study; 4S, Scandanavian Simvastatin Survival Study; LIPID, Long Term Intervention with Pravastatin Trial; AFCAPS/TEXCAPS, Air Force/Texas Atherosclerosis Prevention Study; CARE, Cholesterol and Recurrent Events.

treatment be maximized? Large amounts of basic science data in mammalian species had shown that atherogenesis seemed to *arrest* at an LDL less than 100 mg/dl and appeared to *reverse* at an LDL less than 80 mg/dl. These important basic science observations undergirded several key trials of the twenty-first century.

The first was the seminal 2002 Heart Protection Study (HPS), the largest trial of a statin ever, conducted in 20,536 patients [24]. HPS showed that the largest risk reduction in coronary events occurred in association with the largest reduction in LDL cholesterol. Surprisingly, even patients with supposedly ideal LDL levels at less than 100 mg/dl received huge benefits from statin therapy. Also of high importance: this study included a subgroup of 5,963 patients with diabetes but with no manifest evidence of coronary disease or high cholesterol (mean LDL, 116 mg/dl). The treatment benefit of a 25% risk reduction in coronary events was also extended to these patients with diabetes [24].

Subsequently, the safety and clinical utility of reducing LDL cholesterol levels to even lower values (less than 70 mg/dl) was demonstrated by multiple trials. Chief among these were the 2004 Pravastatin or Atorvastatin Evaluation and Infection-Thrombolysis in Myocardial Infarction 22 Trial (PROVE IT-TIMI 22), the REVERSAL Trial of 2004, the Treat to New Targets (TNT) Trial of 2005, the Incremental Decrease in End-Points Through Aggressive Lipid Lowering (IDEAL) Trial of 2005, and the A Study To Evaluate the Effect of Rosuvastatin on Intravascular Ultrasound Derived Coronary Atheroma Burden (ASTEROID) Trial of 2006 [25–29].

The PROVE IT-TIMI 22 trial enrolled 4162 patients with an acute coronary syndrome; it compared those on standard therapy who had their LDL reduced to less than 100 mg/dl (mean, 95 mg/dl) with 40 mg pravastatin with those given intensive therapy with 80 mg atorvastatin to reduce their LDL to less than 70 md/dl (mean, 62 mg/dl) [25]. The benefit of intensive treatment was demonstrated as early as 30 days of therapy. Mortality from all causes was reduced by 28% in the intensive treatment group, and every other outcome favored the intensive treatment group, except for stroke risk, for which there was little difference.

The REVERSAL trial was a study that demonstrated a reduction in atherosclerosis by ultrasonography in an intensive treatment (LDL less than 80 mg/dl) versus a standard treatment group (LDL less than 100 mg/dl) [26]. The TNT trial was a secondary prevention trial that compared standard treatment (mean LDL, 101 g/dl) with intensive treatment (mean LDL, 77 mg/dl) in patients with stable coronary disease [27]. Once again, superiority of the intensive regimen was demonstrated by an absolute risk reduction of 2.2% and a relative risk reduction of 22% in cardiovascular events in the intensive treatment group versus the standard treatment group.

The IDEAL trial enrolled 8888 patients for secondary prevention. They compared an intensive group that achieved a mean LDL of 81 mg/dl with a standard group with mean LDL of 104 mg/dl [28]. Although major coronary events were not reduced, nonfatal myocardial infarction was reduced in the intensive treatment group.

Finally, Nissen and colleagues undertook another study to directly measure the effects of intensive statin treatment on atherosclerotic plaque burden using intravascular ultrasound in the ASTEROID trial of 2006 [29]. They studied a group in which the LDL cholesterol was reduced from a pretreatment level of 130 mg/dl to a posttreatment level of 60.8 mg/dl with 40 mg/day rosuvastatin. All three direct intravascular measures of atherosclerotic disease burden regressed in just 24 months [29]. Clinical outcomes were not tracked.

How Low Should We Go?

A 2006 meta-analysis combined the results of four major intensive treatment trials (PROVE-IT, TNT, IDEAL, A to Z) to evaluate the evidence in support of more intensive statin therapy to achieve lower LDL cholesterol levels. A total of 27,548 patients were enrolled in the four trials. The meta-analysis revealed a 16% odds reduction in coronary death, myocardial infarction, or any major cardiovascular event [30]. No difference was noted in total or noncardiovascular mortality, but a trend toward decreased cardiovascular mortality was observed [30]. In sum, intensive statin therapy helped to significantly reduce nonfatal cardiovascular events.

Taken as a group, these recent trials of intensive therapy confirm the hypothesis suggested by basic science studies that a lower LDL (less than 80 mg/dl) is superior to an LDL of less than 100 mg/dl by causing a regression of atherosclerosis and a reduction in clinical events across the continuum of cardiovascular disease (Table 1.4). Whether even lower LDL cholesterol levels, that is, less than 60 mg/dl, are safe and beneficial awaits further study. Most experts theorize that there will be an "inflection point" in the risk–benefit curve at some LDL level. Clearly, however, achieving such low cholesterol levels requires an intensity of therapy likely to cost more money, cause more side effects, or trigger noncompliance on the part of patients.

Table 1.4 Results of trials of intensive statin treatment: how low do you go?

	REVERSAL	PROVE-IT	TNT	IDEAL	ASTEROID
Clinical situation	Stable CHD	Acute coronary syndromes	Stable CHD	Prior myocardial infarction	Stable CHD
Outcomes	Ultrasound measure of plaque	Clinical events	Clinical events	Clinical events	Ultrasound measure of plaque
Pretreatment mean LDL (mg/dl)	150	106	152	—	130.4
Posttreatment mean LDL (mg/dl), standard therapy	110	95	101	104	None
Posttreatment mean LDL (mg/dl), intensive therapy	79	62	77	81	60.8
Key results	Reduced plaque burden	28% RR reduction in mortality	22% RR reduction and 2.2% AR reduction in cardiovascular events	Nonfatal myocardial infarction reduced by 12%	Reduced plaque burden

CHD, coronary heart disease; RR, relative risk; AR, absolute risk.

Summary of the Efficacy and Safety of Statin Therapy

Several studies have looked at the safety of statin therapy and have demonstrated no increase in cancer risk or other unexpected complications. In fact, as the decades have progressed, the safety of statin therapy has seemed to be more assured, leading to simvastatin achieving an over-the-counter status in Great Britain in 2004.

Side effects and safety data are reviewed in detail in Chapter 6, but one study deserves special note, that of the Cholesterol Treatment Trialists' (CTT) Collaborators, who published a meta-analysis in 2005 [31]. They reviewed the efficacy and safety data from 14 major statin trials comprising 90,056 patients. They found a 12% reduction in all-cause mortality and a 19% reduction in coronary mortality. Similarly, there were statistically significant reductions in myocardial infarction, in the need for coronary revascularization, and in fatal or nonfatal stroke [31]. Of particular note: they documented that the *proportional reduction in major vascular events achieved differed significantly according to the absolute reduction in LDL cholesterol achieved*. In fact, the absolute benefit of statin treatment was related chiefly to the absolute reduction in LDL cholesterol achieved. Lower LDL proved to be better.

Safety was demonstrated by showing that there was no evidence that statins increased the incidence of cancer at any site or cancer incidence overall in the group receiving therapy with statins for elevated cholesterol [31]. Additionally, the 5-year excess risk for rhabdomyolysis was not significant for the statin-treated group versus the control group.

Evidence Summary for Primary Prevention

The evidence supporting the utility of the primary prevention of atherosclerotic disease is variable, depending upon the level of cardiac risk in the patient. By stratifying patients into three risk categories—low (less than 0.6% annual incidence), medium (0.6% to less than 1.4% annual incidence), and high (greater than 1.5% annual incidence)—for coronary heart disease, general evidence-based statements can be made based on the work by the *British Medical Journal* [32].

No studies of primary prevention have been conducted in patients at *low risk*. Therefore, the risks and benefits are unknown. For patients at *medium risk*, fibrates are beneficial, and resins and statins are likely to be beneficial in reducing coronary heart disease risk. For patients at *high risk*, statins are beneficial. No studies were found that used fibrates, niacin, or resins in this subgroup [32].

Evidence Summary for Secondary Prevention

The evidence in support of the secondary prevention of atherosclerotic vascular disease by the treatment of hyperlipidemia is quite broad. In fact, multiple, nonspecific lipid-lowering treatments reduce overall mortality, cardiovascular mortality, and nonfatal cardiovascular events when compared with not lowering cholesterol

[33]. Statins are clearly beneficial, and this benefit extends to both genders and to the elderly. Fibrates are likely to be beneficial in secondary prevention.

Nondrug treatments were also examined in a thorough evidence review for the secondary prevention of cardiovascular disease [33]. Exercise is beneficial. Psychological treatment to reduce stress, a Mediterranean diet, and smoking cessation are all likely to be beneficial. Advice to eat less fat, to eat more fiber, or to consume more fish oil still is of unknown effectiveness because of the small number of studies. In contrast, antioxidant vitamins, multivitamins, and vitamin C are unlikely to be beneficial, and beta-carotene and vitamin E are likely to be harmful [33].

The American Heart Association and the American College of Cardiology (AHA/ACC) issued evidence-based guidelines in 2006 for the secondary prevention of atherosclerotic vascular disease that grade the evidence in support of all possible treatment modalities. In particular, they added the recent trial information on the intensive treatment of dyslipidemia to LDL cholesterol levels of less than 70 mg/dl to their guidelines. The guidelines provide an excellent summary using traditional AHA evidence classification of recommendations: Class I (effective), Class II (possibly effective), and Class III (harmful). They also grade the evidence:

Table 1.5 Summary of the 2006 American Heart Association and the American College of Cardiology (AHA/ACC) recommendations for the secondary prevention of atherosclerotic vascular disease

Intervention	Recommendations	Level of evidence
Smoking cessation	Assist with a plan for quitting	I (B)
Blood pressure control	Goal less than 140/90 mm Hg or less than 130/80 mm Hg for those with diabetes or chronic kidney disease	I (A)
Lipid management	For all, LDL less than 100 mg/dl and reduction to an LDL level less than 70 mg/dl is reasonable	I (A) II (A)
Physical activity	30 to 60 min/day for 5 to 7 days per week	I (B)
Weight management	Maintain BMI 18.5 to 24.9 kg/m[2] and waist less than 40 in. in men and less than 35 in. in women	I (B)
Diabetes management	Maintain hemoglobin A1c less than 7.0%	I (B)
Antiplatelet therapy	Start aspirin 75–162 mg/day unless contraindicated	I (A)
Renin-angiotensin system blockers	Start and continue ACE inhibitors or ARBs in patients with LV ejection fraction less than 40%	I (A)
Beta-blockers	Start and continue for any patients who have had an acute coronary syndrome or LV dysfunction	I (A)
Influenza vaccination	Annual vaccination	I (B)

BMI, body mass index; ACE, angiotensin-converting enzyme; ARB, angiotensin receptor blocker; LV, left ventricular.
Source: Data from Smith SC, Allen J, Blair SN, et al. AHA/ACC guidelines for secondary prevention for patients with coronary and other atherosclerotic vascular disease: 2006 update. Circulation 2006;113:2363–2372 [34].

A (multiple randomized controlled trials or meta-analyses), B (single randomized trial or multiple nonrandomized trials), or C (expert opinion, case studies, or standard of care). Their recommendations, which are very extensive, are summarized in Table 1.5 [34].

References

1. Ross R. Atherosclerosis: an inflammatory disease. N Engl J Med 1999;340:115–126.
2. Forrester JS. Prevention of plaque rupture: a new paradigm of therapy. Ann Intern Med 2002;137:823–833.
3. Kavey RW, Daniels SR, Lauer RM, et al. American Heart Association Guidelines for primary prevention of atherosclerotic cardiovascular disease beginning in childhood. Circulation 2003;107:1562–1566.
4. Anonymous. Relationship of atherosclerosis in young men to serum lipoprotein cholesterol concentrations and smoking: a preliminary report from the Pathobiological Determinants of Atherosclerosis in Youth (PDAY) Research Group. JAMA 1990;264:3018–3024.
5. Mahoney LT, Burns TL, Stanford W, et al. Coronary risk factors measured in childhood and young adult life are associated with coronary artery calcification in young adults: the Muscatine Study. J Am Coll Cardiol 1996;27:277–284.
6. Berenson GS, Srinivasan SR, Bao W, et al. Association between multiple cardiovascular risk factors and atherosclerosis in children and young adults: the Bogalusa Heart Study. N Engl J Med 1998;338:1650–1656.
7. Li S, Chen W, Srinivasan SR, et al. Childhood cardiovascular risk factors and carotid vascular changes in adulthood. JAMA 2003;290:2271–2277.
8. Obarzanek E, Kimm SY, Barton BA, et al. Long-term safety and efficacy of a cholesterol-lowering diet in children with elevated LDL cholesterol: seven year results of the Dietary Intervention Study in Children (DISC). Pediatrics 2001;107:256–264.
9. Flynn BS, Warden JK, Secker-Walker R. Cigarette smoking prevention: effects of mass media and school interventions. J Health Educ 1995;26:545–551.
10. Sallis JF, McKenzie TL, Alcarez JE, et al. The effects of a 2-year physical education program (SPARK) on physical activity and fitness in elementary school students. Am J Public Health 1997;87:1328–1334.
11. Stein EA, Illingsworth DR, Kwiterovich PO, et al. Efficacy and safety of lovastatin in adolescent males with heterozygous familial hypercholesterolemia: a randomized controlled trial. JAMA 1999;281:137–144.
12. Wiegman A, Hutten BA, Groot ED, et al. Efficacy and safety of statin therapy in children with familial hypercholesterolemia. JAMA 2004;292:331–337.
13. Anonymous. The Lipid Research Clinics Coronary Primary Prevention Trial results. JAMA 1984;251(3):351–364.
14. Blankenhorn DH, Nessim SA, Johnson RL, et al. Beneficial effects of combined colestipol-niacin therapy on coronary atherosclerosis and coronary venous bypass grafts. JAMA 1987;257(23):3233–3240.
15. Frick MH, Elo O, Haapa K, et al. Helsinki Heart Study. N Engl J Med 1987;317:1237–1245.
16. Anonymous. WHO cooperative trial on primary prevention of ischaemic heart disease with clofibrate to lower serum cholesterol: final mortality follow-up. Lancet 1984;2:600–604.
17. Shepherd J, Cobbe SM, Ford I, et al. Prevention of coronary heart disease with pravastatin in men with hypercholesterolemia. West of Scotland Coronary Prevention Study Group. N Engl J Med 1995;333:1301–1307.
18. Downs JR, Clearfield M, Weis S, et al. Primary prevention of acute coronary events with lovastatin in men and women with average cholesterol levels. Results of AFCAPS/TEXCAPS. JAMA 1998;279:1615–1622.

19. Scandanavian Simvastatin Survival Study Group. Randomized trial of cholesterol lowering in 4444 patients with coronary heart disease: the Scandinavian Simvastatin Survival Study (4S). Lancet 1994;344:1383–1389.
20. The Lipid Study Group. LIPID (Long-Term Intervention with Pravastatin in Ischemic Disease) Study: a randomized trial in patients with previous acute myocardial infarction and/or unstable angina pectoris. Am J Cardiol 1995;76:474–479.
21. Sacks FM, Pfeffer MA, Moye LA, et al. The effect of pravastatin on coronary events after myocardial infarction in patients with average cholesterol levels. Cholesterol and Recurrent Events Trial Investigators. N Engl J Med 1996;335:1001–1009.
22. Robins SJ, Collins D, Wittes JT, et al. Relation of gemfibrozil treatment and lipid levels with major coronary events. VA-HIT: a randomized controlled trial. JAMA 2001;285;1585–1591.
23. Schwartz GG, Olsson AG, Ezekowitz MD, et al. Effects of atorvastatin on early recurrent ischemic events in acute coronary syndromes. The MIRACL study: a randomized controlled trial. JAMA 2001;285:1711–1718.
24. Anonymous. MRC/BHF Heart Protection Study of cholesterol-lowering with simvastatin in 5963 people with diabetes: a randomized placebo-controlled trial. Lancet 2003;361: 2005–2015.
25. Cannon CP, Braunwald E, McCabe CH, et al. Comparison of intensive and moderate lipid lowering with statins after acute coronary syndromes. N Engl J Med 2004;350:1495–1504.
26. Nissen SE, Tuzcu EM, Schoenhagen P, et al. Effect of intensive compared with moderate lipid-lowering therapy on progression of coronary atherosclerosis: a randomized controlled trial. JAMA 2004;291:1071–1080.
27. LaRosa JC, Grundy SM, Waters DD, et al. Intensive lipid lowering with atorvastatin in patients with stable coronary disease. N Engl J Med 2005;352:1425–1435.
28. Pedersen TR, Faergeman O, Kastelein JJP, et al. High-dose atorvastatin vs. usual-dose simvastatin for secondary prevention after myocardial infarction. IDEAL study: a randomized controlled trial. JAMA 2005;294:2437–2445.
29. Nissen SE, Nicholls SJ, Sipahi I, et al. Effect of very high-intensity statin therapy on regression of coronary atherosclerosis: the ASTEROID trial. JAMA 2006;295:1556–1565.
30. Cannon CP, Steinberg BA, Murphy SA, et al. Meta-analysis of cardiovascular outcomes trials comparing intensive versus moderate statin therapy. J Am Coll Cardiol 2006;48:438–445.
31. Anonymous. Efficacy and safety of cholesterol lowering treatment: prospective meta-analysis of data from 90,056 participants in 14 randomized trials of statins. Lancet 2005;366: 1267–1277.
32. Pignone M. Primary prevention: dyslipidemia. In: British Medical Journal. Clinical evidence, 15th edn. London: BMJ Publishing Group, 2006:38–40.
33. Gami A. Secondary prevention of ischemic cardiac events. In: British Medical Journal. Clinical evidence, 15th edn. London: BMJ Publishing Group, 2006:43–48.
34. Smith SC, Allen J, Blair SN, et al. AHA/ACC guidelines for secondary prevention for patients with coronary and other atherosclerotic vascular disease: 2006 update. Circulation 2006;113:2363–2372.

Suggested Key Readings

Cannon CP, Steinberg BA, Murphy SA, et al. Meta-analysis of cardiovascular outcomes trials comparing intensive versus moderate statin therapy. J Am Coll Cardiol 2006;48:438–445.
Forrester JS. Prevention of plaque rupture: a new paradigm of therapy. Ann Intern Med 2002;137:823–833.
Smith SC, Allen J, Blair SN, et al. AHA/ACC guidelines for secondary prevention for patients with coronary and other atherosclerotic vascular disease: 2006 update. Circulation 2006;113: 2363–2372.

Chapter 2
National Cholesterol Education Program: Adult Treatment Panel III Guidelines and the 2004 Update

James W. Haynes and Erika V. Barger

Introduction

The Third Report of the Expert Panel on Detection, Evaluation, and Treatment of High Blood Cholesterol in Adults [Adult Treatment Panel III (ATP III)] was published in 2002 and provided updated guidelines for cholesterol measurement and management [1]. This National Cholesterol Education Program was updated with further recommendations in 2004 [2]. This chapter reviews the major recommendations made in each document and provides a level of evidence corresponding to those recommendations. Table 2.1 outlines the level of evidence designation used throughout the report.

ATP made it very clear that its report should not be viewed as a standard of practice but that "evidence derived from empirical data can lead to generalities for guiding practice, but such guidance need not hold for individual patients" [3].

Summary

ATP III was consistent with ATP I and ATP II by providing recommendations regarding the clinical management of elevated cholesterol levels. For patients with elevated low density lipoprotein (LDL) or borderline high LDL cholesterol levels plus two major risk factors, ATP I provided a framework for primary prevention of cardiovascular disease [4]. ATP II confirmed its predecessor's approach and added the intensive management of LDL cholesterol in patients with recognized coronary heart disease (CHD) [5]. For these patients with known CHD, ATP II set a goal LDL of less than 100 mg/dl. While ATP III continued the focus on elevated LDL levels as the primary target of therapy, it called for a more-rigorous LDL-lowering goal in CHD patients and CHD equivalents. In addition, ATP III recommended paying

---

J.W. Haynes
Program Director, Headquarters Air Armament Center Family Medicine Residency, Department of Family Medicine, Eglin Air Force Base Hospital, FL

B.V. Reamy (ed.), *Hyperlipidemia Management for Primary Care*,
DOI: 10.1007/978-0-387-76606-5_2, © Springer Science+Business Media, LLC 2008

Table 2.1 Type of evidence

Type of Evidence:	
Category of type of evidence	Description of type of evidence
A	Major randomized controlled clinical trials (RCTs)
B	Smaller RCTs and meta-analyses of other clinical trials
C	Observational and metabolic studies
D	Clinical experience
Strength of Evidence:	
Category of strength of evidence	Description of strength of evidence
1	Very strong evidence
2	Moderately strong evidence
3	Strong trend

Source: Adapted with permission from National Cholesterol Education Program (NCEP) Expert Panel on Detection, Evaluation, and Treatment of High Blood Cholesterol in Adults (Adult Treatment Panel III). Third Report of the National Cholesterol Education Program (NCEP) Expert Panel on Detection, Evaluation, and Treatment of High Blood Cholesterol in Adults (Adult Treatment Panel III) final report. Circulation 2002;106:3143–3421.

increased attention to preventing CHD in those patients without identifiable coronary disease yet with multiple risk factors. The major recommendations made by this report, with their corresponding levels of evidence, are captured in Table 2.2. Tables 2.3 and 2.4 highlight the updated features of ATP III when compared to its predecessor, ATP II. Table 2.5 denotes ATP III recommended normal lipid values.

Risk Assessment

Based on the principle of risk-reduction therapy, the 2002 report recommended establishing an absolute risk quotient for each patient before determining optimal therapy. This risk assessment combines a lipoprotein analysis and the identification and quantification of other cardiac risk factors. It also recommended classifying a patient into risk categories based on their baseline LDL level (refer to normal lipid values) and obtaining a fasting lipoprotein profile every 5 years in all adults 20 years old and older. The three risk categories recommended were CHD and CHD risk equivalents (10-year risk for CHD greater than 20%); multiple (2+) risk factors (10-year risk, 20% or less); and zero to one risk factor (10-year risk less than 10%). This classification ultimately determines optimal LDL levels (Table 2.6) and leads to recommended therapeutic interventions to lower LDL if needed. The report also labeled individuals with multiple risk factors that have more than a 20% risk for major coronary events within 10 years despite not having CHD as "CHD equivalents" (C1) [6]. CHD equivalents included those patients with other forms of atherosclerotic disease (peripheral arterial disease, abdominal aortic aneurysm, symptomatic carotid artery disease), diabetes, and/or those with multiple risk factors that add up to a 10-year risk greater than 20%. Quantification of CHD risk status is determined using the Framingham risk score obtained by using Table 2.7 for men and Table 2.8 for women. PDA versions of the risk score

Table 2.2 Key Adult Treatment Panel (ATP) III findings/recommendations with evidence basis

LDL cholesterol should continue to be the primary target of cholesterol-lowering therapy	A1, B1,C1
Persons without identifiable coronary disease but with multiple risk factors should be considered for primary preventive LDL-lowering therapy	A1, B1
Routine cholesterol testing should begin in young adulthood (at 20 years of age or older)	C1
A low HDL cholesterol level is strongly and inversely associated with risk for coronary heart disease (CHD)	C1
Primary management of metabolic syndrome should be to reverse root causes (overweight/obesity/physical inactivity) and other modifiable risk factors	C1
Persons with established CHD should receive intensive LDL-lowering therapy	A1, A2 B1, C1
Persons with established CHD who have a baseline LDL cholesterol of 130 mg/dl or higher should be started on lipid-lowering drugs simultaneously with TLC therapy	A1
When 10-year risk for hard CHD is less than 10%, LDL-lowering drugs should be used judiciously because of limited cost-effectiveness	A2
When 10-year risk for hard CHD is 10%–20%, LDL-lowering drugs carry an acceptable cost-effectiveness	B1
For persons without identifiable CHD but with multiple risk factors, their LDL level should be maintained at less than 130 mg/dl	A1
In primary prevention, consider LDL-lowering drugs for patients whose 10-year risk is less than 10% and whose LDL is 160 mg/dl or higher despite adequate lifestyle change	A1, B1
In primary prevention, consider LDL-lowering drugs in patients whose 10-year risk is 10%–20% and whose LDL is 130 mg/dl or higher despite adequate lifestyle changes	A1, B1
In primary prevention, a LDL goal of less than 100 mg/dl in patients whose 10-year risk is greater than 20%	A1, B1
Persons with type 2 diabetes should be managed as a CHD risk equivalent; treatment for LDL cholesterol should follow recommendations for persons with established CHD	A2, C1
Persons with clinical forms of noncoronary atherosclerosis should have the same LDL goals as those for persons with established CHD	C1
Use of a multidisciplinary team to manage patients with high serum cholesterol	A2
Statins should be considered first-line drugs when LDL-lowering drugs are indicated to achieve LDL treatment goals	A1

Source: Adapted with permission from National Cholesterol Education Program (NCEP) Expert Panel on Detection, Evaluation, and Treatment of High Blood Cholesterol in Adults (Adult Treatment Panel III). Third Report of the National Cholesterol Education Program (NCEP) Expert Panel on Detection, Evaluation, and Treatment of High Blood Cholesterol in Adults (Adult Treatment Panel III) final report. Circulation 2002;106:3143–3421.

calculator can be downloaded from the National Heart, Lung and Blood Institute website athp2010.nhlbihin.net/atpiii/atp3palm.htm.

Risk Assessment Basics

The first step to calculating a Framingham CHD risk score is to determine the number of risk factors present (age, total cholesterol level, smoking status, high

Table 2.3 Shared features of ATP III and ATP II

- Continued identification of LDL cholesterol lowering as the primary goal of therapy
- Consideration of high LDL cholesterol (160 mg/dl or more) as a potential target for LDL-lowering drug therapy, specifically as follows:
    - For persons with multiple risk factors whose LDL levels are high (160 mg/dl or higher) after dietary therapy, consideration of drug therapy is recommended
    - For persons with 0–1 risk factor, consideration of drug therapy (after dietary therapy) is optional for LDL 160–189 mg/dl and recommended for LDL 190 mg/dl or higher
- Emphasis on intensive LDL-lowering therapy in persons with established CHD
- Identification of three categories of risk for different LDL goals and different intensities of LDL-lowering therapy:
    - CHD and CHD risk equivalents (other forms of clinical atherosclerotic disease)
    - Multiple (2+) risk factors
    - 0–1 risk factor
- Identification of subpopulations besides middle-aged men for detection of high LDL cholesterol (and other lipid risk factors) and for clinical intervention; these include:
    - Young adults
    - Postmenopausal women
    - Postmenopausal women
    - Older persons
- Emphasis on weight loss and physical activity to enhance risk reduction in persons with elevated LDL cholesterol

Source: Adapted with permission from National Cholesterol Education Program (NCEP) Expert Panel on Detection, Evaluation, and Treatment of High Blood Cholesterol in Adults (Adult Treatment Panel III). Third Report of the National Cholesterol Education Program (NCEP) Expert Panel on Detection, Evaluation, and Treatment of High Blood Cholesterol in Adults (Adult Treatment Panel III) final report. Circulation 2002;106:3143–3421.

density lipoprotein (HDL) cholesterol level, and systolic blood pressure reading). Patients with two or more risk factors then undergo risk assessment using the Framingham scoring tables noted earlier to identify persons with an elevated 10-year risk. Note that LDL cholesterol level is not used as a risk factor because it is the target of therapy. Initial assessments require values for total cholesterol and HDL whereas optimal risk scoring utilizes the average of at least two lipoprotein analysis measurements. The blood pressure value (a major independent risk factor for CHD) used is the one taken at the time of the risk assessment regardless of the presence or absence of antihypertensive therapy. An extra point is added to the risk score if the patient is on antihypertensive therapy. Smoking (another strong, independent risk factor for CHD) points are determined by whether the patient has smoked any cigarettes in the preceding month. The points of each risk category are combined, and an absolute 10-year risk is determined using the embedded estimate tables.

The benefit of using the risk scoring system is that it allows better identification of patients requiring intensive treatment based on risk category assignment. When patients have zero or one risk factor, ATP III recommends not performing the Framingham risk factor scoring because the 10-year risk seldom reaches levels for intensive therapy to be considered. The 2002 report defines the initial computation of 10-year risk score as the patient's "core risk status." Only after the core risk status has been determined should other risk modifiers be taken into account for therapeutic decision making.

Table 2.4 New features of ATP III

Focus on Multiple Risk Factors

- Raises persons with diabetes without CHD, most of whom display multiple risk factors, to the risk level of CHD risk equivalent
- Uses Framingham projections of 10-year absolute CHD risk (i.e., the percent probability of having a CHD event in 10 years) to identify certain patients with multiple (2+) risk factors for more intensive treatment
- Identifies persons with multiple metabolic risk factors (metabolic syndrome) as candidates for intensified therapeutic lifestyle changes

Modifications of Lipid and Lipoprotein Classification

- Identifies LDL cholesterol less than 100 mg/dl as optimal
- Raises categorical low HDL cholesterol from less than 35 mg/dl to less than 40 mg/dl because the latter is a better measure of a depressed HDL
- Lowers the triglyceride classification cutpoints to give more attention to moderate elevations

Support for Implementation

- Recommends a complete lipoprotein profile (total cholesterol, LDL cholesterol, HDL cholesterol, and triglycerides) as the preferred initial test, rather than screening for total cholesterol and HDL alone
- Encourages use of plant stanols/sterols and viscous (soluble) fiber as therapeutic dietary options to enhance lowering of LDL cholesterol
- Presents strategies for promoting adherence to therapeutic lifestyle changes and drug therapies
- Recommends treatment beyond LDL lowering for persons with triglycerides 200 mg/dl or higher

Source: Adapted with permission from National Cholesterol Education Program (NCEP) Expert Panel on Detection, Evaluation, and Treatment of High Blood Cholesterol in Adults (Adult Treatment Panel III). Third Report of the National Cholesterol Education Program (NCEP) Expert Panel on Detection, Evaluation, and Treatment of High Blood Cholesterol in Adults (Adult Treatment Panel III) final report. Circulation 2002;106:3143–3421.

Table 2.5 ATP III normal lipid values

LDL cholesterol	
Less than 100	Optimal
100–129	Near optimal/above optimal
130–159	Borderline high
160–189	High
More than 190	Very high
Total cholesterol	
Less than 200	Desirable
200–239	Borderline high
More than 240	High
HDL cholesterol	
Less than 40	Low
More than 60	High

Source: Adapted with permission from National Cholesterol Education Program (NCEP) Expert Panel on Detection, Evaluation, and Treatment of High Blood Cholesterol in Adults (Adult Treatment Panel III). Third Report of the National Cholesterol Education Program (NCEP) Expert Panel on Detection, Evaluation, and Treatment of High Blood Cholesterol in Adults (Adult Treatment Panel III) final report. Circulation 2002;106:3143–3421.

Table 2.6 Three categories of risk that modify LDL cholesterol goals

Risk category	LDL goal (mg/dl)
CHD and CHD risk equivalents	Less than 100
Multiple (2+) risk factors	Less than 130
Zero or 1 risk factor	Less than 160

Source: Adapted with permission from National Cholesterol Education Program (NCEP) Expert Panel on Detection, Evaluation, and Treatment of High Blood Cholesterol in Adults (Adult Treatment Panel III). Third Report of the National Cholesterol Education Program (NCEP) Expert Panel on Detection, Evaluation, and Treatment of High Blood Cholesterol in Adults (Adult Treatment Panel III) final report. Circulation 2002;106:3143–3421.

Table 2.7 Estimate of 10-year risk for men (Framingham Point Scores)

Age	Points
20–34	−9
35–39	−4
40–44	0
45–49	3
50–54	6
55–59	8
60–64	10
65–69	11
70–74	12
75–79	13

Total Cholesterol	Points				
	Age 20–39	Age 40–49	Age 50–59	Age 60–69	Age 70–79
<160	0	0	0	0	0
160–199	4	3	2	1	0
200–239	7	5	3	1	0
240–279	9	6	4	2	1
>280	11	8	5	3	1

	Points				
	Age 20–39	Age 40–49	Age 50–59	Age 60–69	Age 70–79
Nonsmoker	0	0	0	0	0
Smoker	8	5	3	1	1

HDL (mg/dl)	Points
> 60	−1
50–59	0
40–49	1
<40	2

Systolic BP (mmHg)	If Untreated	If treated
<120	0	0
120–129	0	1
130–139	1	2
140–159	1	2
>160	2	3

Table 2.7 (continued)

Point Total	10-Year Risk (%)
<0	<1
0	1
1	1
2	1
3	1
4	1
5	2
6	2
7	3
8	4
9	5
10	6
11	8
12	10
13	12
14	16
15	20
16	25
>17	>30

Source: Adapted with permission from National Cholesterol Education Program (NCEP) Expert Panel on Detection, Evaluation, and Treatment of High Blood Cholesterol in Adults (Adult Treatment Panel III). Third Report of the National Cholesterol Education Program (NCEP) Expert Panel on Detection, Evaluation, and Treatment of High Blood Cholesterol in Adults (Adult Treatment Panel III) final report. Circulation 2002;106:3143–3421.

Other Risk Factors

ATP III acknowledged the influence of other risk factors in the development of CHD. It categorizes these other risk factors as life habit risk factors and emerging lipid and emerging nonlipid factors. Obesity, physical inactivity, and atherogenic diet were all recognized as life habit risk factors. Additionally, ATP III recognized triglycerides and lipoprotein remnants as significant emerging lipid risk factors while noting lipoprotein(a), small LDL particles, HDL subspecies, apolipoprotein B, and apolipoprotein A-1 as potential future lipid risk factors. Emerging nonlipid risk factors noted by ATP III include homocysteine, prothrombotic and proinflammatory factors, impaired fasting glucose, and evidence of subclinical atherosclerotic disease (peripheral arterial disease, abnormal EKGs, myocardial perfusion imaging, and stress echocardiography, carotid intimal medial thickening, and coronary calcium). This guideline recognized the need to target life habit risk factors but does not use these to set lower goals of LDL cholesterol therapy. Similarly, ATP III recognized that the emerging risk factors play a role in CHD development and can have a part in modifying therapeutic decisions, but it did not factor these risk factors into setting LDL cholesterol targets.

Metabolic Syndrome

ATP III recognized that the presence of metabolic syndrome accentuated the risk of CHD when coupled with the presence of elevated LDL cholesterol. This syndrome is characterized by abdominal obesity, atherogenic dyslipidemia, elevated blood pressure, insulin resistance, and prothrombotic and proinflammatory states. The presence of three of five of the determinants in Table 2.9 is thought to be diagnostic for metabolic syndrome.

The report endorsed therapeutic lifestyle changes (TLC) as first-line therapy for metabolic syndrome, with an emphasis on weight loss and adequate exercise as well as aggressive treatment of elevated triglycerides (see Table 2.2 for evidence ratings).

Table 2.8 Estimate of 10-year risk for women (Framingham Point Scores)

Age	Points
20–34	−7
35–39	−3
40–44	0
45–49	3
50–54	6
55–59	8
60–64	10
65–69	12
70–74	14
75–79	16

Total Cholesterol	Points				
	Age 20–39	Age 40–49	Age 50–59	Age 60–69	Age 70–79
<160	0	0	0	0	0
160–199	4	3	2	1	1
200–239	8	6	4	2	1
240–279	11	8	5	3	2
>280	13	10	7	4	2

	Points				
	Age 20–39	Age 40–49	Age 50–59	Age 60–69	Age 70–79
Nonsmoker	0	0	0	0	0
Smoker	9	7	4	2	1

HDL (mg/dl)	Points
>60	−1
50–59	0
40–49	1
<40	2

Systolic BP (mmHg)	If Untreated	If Untreated
<120	0	0
120–129	1	3
130–139	2	4
140–159	3	5
>160	4	6

Table 2.8 (continued)

Point Total	10-Year Risk (%)
<9	<1
9	1
10	1
11	1
12	1
13	2
14	2
15	3
16	4
17	5
18	6
19	8
20	11
21	14
22	17
23	22
24	27
>25	>30

Source: Adapted with permission from National Cholesterol Education Program (NCEP) Expert Panel on Detection, Evaluation, and Treatment of High Blood Cholesterol in Adults (Adult Treatment Panel III). Third Report of the National Cholesterol Education Program (NCEP) Expert Panel on Detection, Evaluation, and Treatment of High Blood Cholesterol in Adults (Adult Treatment Panel III) final report. Circulation 2002;106:3143–3421.

Cost-Effectiveness and Risk Assessment

This 2002 panel report appreciated the fact that LDL-lowering medications are a major expense and may not be cost effective using then-current economic efficiency standards. It also recognized that LDL-lowering drug therapy was highly cost effective in persons with established CHD and for primary prevention in patients at high risk. Additionally, ATP III stated that when 10-year risk for hard CHD [myocardial infarction (MI) + CHD death] was 10% to 20% per year, LDL-lowering drug therapy was cost effective compared to most other medical interventions. Additionally, it stated that when 10-year risk for hard CHD was less than 10% per year, LDL-lowering drug therapy exceeded cost-effectiveness standards. Based on these findings, the report recommended judicious use of LDL-lowering drugs if 10-year risk was less than 10%, noting that diet therapy was much more cost effective.

Finally, ATP III recommended that LDL-lowering medications should be considered if LDL cholesterol levels remained at 160 mg/dl or higher after a diet therapy trial in patients with a 10-year risk less than 10% and multiple major risk factors. It also acknowledged that the need to reduce long-term risk can override the need to stay within cost-effectiveness criteria (see Table 2.2 for evidence ratings).

Table 2.9 Clinical identification of the metabolic syndrome[a]

Risk factor	Defining level
Abdominal obesity	Waist circumference[b]
Men	>102 cm (>40 in.)
Women	>88 cm (>35 in.)
Triglycerides	≥150 mg/dl
HDL cholesterol	
Men	<40 mg/dl
Women	<50 mg/dl
Blood pressure	≥130/85 mmHg
Fasting glucose	≥110 mg/dl

[a]The ATP III panel did not find adequate evidence to recommend routine measurement of insulin resistance (e.g., plasma insulin), proinflammatory state (e.g., high-sensitivity C-reactive protein), or prothrombotic state (e.g., fibrinogen or PAI-1) in the diagnosis of metabolic syndrome.

[b]Some male persons can develop multiple metabolic risk factors when the waist circumference is only marginally increased, e.g., 94–102 cm (37–39 in.). Such persons may have a strong genetic contribution to insulin resistance. They should benefit from changes in life habits, similarly to men with categorical increases in waist circumference.

Source: Adapted with permission from National Cholesterol Education Program (NCEP) Expert Panel on Detection, Evaluation, and Treatment of High Blood Cholesterol in Adults (Adult Treatment Panel III). Third Report of the National Cholesterol Education Program (NCEP) Expert Panel on Detection, Evaluation, and Treatment of High Blood Cholesterol in Adults (Adult Treatment Panel III) final report. Circulation 2002;106:3143–3421.

Primary Prevention with LDL-Lowering Therapy

ATP III endorsed a public health approach to primary prevention of CHD, which consisted of lifestyle changes including (1) reduced intake of saturated fat and cholesterol, (2) increased physical activity, and (3) weight control. Primary prevention LDL goals rested on a patient's absolute risk of CHD where higher risk leads to lower recommended goals. Regardless of risk, recent primary prevention trials as outlined in Chapter 1 clearly showed that LDL-lowering medications decreased the risk for CHD events and death in the short term (less than 10 years) and the long term (over a lifetime). The major primary prevention recommendations and evidence ratings are listed in Table 2.2.

Level A1 and B1 evidence also supported the following recommendations. (1) Efforts should be made to reduce LDL cholesterol in low-risk patients (0–1 risk factors) to less than 160 mg/dl and that lifestyle changes should be stressed when levels are 130 to 159 mg/dl; (2) drug therapy should be avoided in the aforementioned patients because of the lack of safety data and low cost-effectiveness ratios; (3) LDL-lowering drugs should be considered when LDL cholesterol levels are borderline (160–189 mg/dl) and strongly encouraged when 190 mg/dl or higher if lifestyle changes are inadequate; and (4) use of LDL-lowering medication therapy

should be considered for patients with zero to one major risk factors, LDL cholesterol level in the 160–189 mg/dl range, and an additional severe single risk factor,
a significant family history of premature CHD, or the presence of emerging risk or
life habit factors.

This 2002 panel also recommended: (1) routine cholesterol screening for all
adults 20 years of age or older; (2) promoting lifestyle modification measures
for these young adults with LDL cholesterol levels between 100 and 129 mg/dl;
(3) instituting lifestyle changes in these young adults with a LDL cholesterol
level between 130 and 159 mg/dl; (4) expanding clinical attention to include TLC
implementation in young adults with a LDL cholesterol level between 160 and
189 mg/dl with consideration for LDL-lowering medication use if TLC fails; and
(5) considering LDL-lowering drugs for those young adults with a LDL cholesterol
of 190 mg/dl or higher when TLC fails.

ATP III also recommended that all patients with an elevated LDL cholesterol
level undergo a workup to rule out secondary dyslipidemias. The major causes of
these secondary maladies include diabetes, hypothyroidism, nephrotic syndrome,
obstructive liver disease, chronic renal failure, and specific medication use
[progestins, anabolic steroids, corticosteroids, and human immunodeficiency virus
(HIV)-related protease inhibitors].

Secondary Prevention with LDL-Lowering Therapy

Clinical trials preceding ATP III demonstrated that LDL-lowering interventions
reduced total mortality, coronary mortality, major coronary events, coronary artery
procedures, and strokes in persons with known CHD. The three main studies that
produced these results were the 4S, the CARE, and the LIPID studies outlined
in Chapter 1. Hence, this panel set an LDL cholesterol goal of 100 mg/dl or less
as the target for secondary prevention of CHD in these patients and applied this
goal to those patients with CHD risk equivalents as well. This recommendation was
supported by evidence that revealed LDL cholesterol lowering significantly reduced
risk for recurrent major CHD events. Furthermore, the report recognized evidence
that the 10-year risk for major coronary events in a person with diabetes mellitus
(DM) type 2 approximated the risk of a patient with established CHD. It also noted
that some type I diabetics, while having a slightly lower 10-year risk for developing
CHD, clearly have a high long-term risk of major coronary events. This evidence led
ATP III contributors to establish similar LDL cholesterol-lowering goals for type II
diabetics and those patients with established CHD.

LDL-Lowering Therapy in Three Risk Categories

Therapeutic lifestyle changes (TLC) and drug therapy comprise the major treatment
arms to lower LDL cholesterol. Table 2.10, adapted from ATP III, defines the LDL

Table 2. 10 LDL cholesterol goals and cutpoints for therapeutic lifestyle changes (TLC) and drug therapy in different risk categories

Risk category	LDL goal	LDL level at which to initiate TLC	LDL level at which consider drug therapy
CHD or CHD risk equivalents (10-year risk >20%)	<100 mg/dl	≥100 mg/dl	≥130 mg/dl (100–129 mg/dl; drug optional)[a]
2+ risk factors (10-year risk ≤20%)	<130 mg/dl	≥130 mg/dl	10-year risk 10%–20%: ≥130 mg/dl
0–1 risk factor[b]	<160 mg/dl	≥160 mg/dl	10-year risk <10%: ≥160 mg/dl ≥190 mg/dl (160–189 mg/dl: LDL-lowering drug optional)

[a]Some authorities recommend use of LDL-lowering drugs in this category if an LDL cholesterol less than 100 mg/dl cannot be achieved by TLCs. Others prefer use of drugs that primarily modify triglycerides and HDL, e.g., nicotinic acid or fibrate. Clinical judgment also may call for deferring drug therapy in this subcategory.

[b]Almost all patients with 0–1 risk factor have a 10-year risk less than 10%; thus, 10-year risk factor assessment not necessary.

Source: Adapted with permission from National Cholesterol Education Program (NCEP) Expert Panel on Detection, Evaluation, and Treatment of High Blood Cholesterol in Adults (Adult Treatment Panel III). Third Report of the National Cholesterol Education Program (NCEP) Expert Panel on Detection, Evaluation, and Treatment of High Blood Cholesterol in Adults (Adult Treatment Panel III) final report. Circulation 2002;106:3143–3421.

cholesterol goals for the three levels of risk as well as giving recommendations for starting TLC and considering drug therapy based on the risk category.

Therapeutic Lifestyle Changes in LDL-Lowering Therapy

The salient elements of the therapeutic lifestyle changes (TLC) recommended by ATP III include dietary changes (including the use of augmenting plant stanols/sterols and increased soluble fiber to lower LDL cholesterol), weight loss, and increased physical activity. Table 2.11 gives the dietary composition recommended in the report. Once maximum reduction of LDL cholesterol is achieved with dietary measures, the report recommends shifting treatment emphasis to the management of metabolic syndrome and its related lipid risk factors (high triglycerides/low HDL). Figure 2.1 illustrates a recommended model for instituting TLC. The diet recommendations of the report are made secondary to the fact that a higher intake of mostly unsaturated fat can help reduce triglycerides and raise HDL in patients with metabolic syndrome. ATP III emphasizes that weight loss helps both lipid and nonlipid risk factors in overweight and obese patients.

It should be noted that the report encouraged clinicians to use registered dieticians or other nutritionists to enhance *medical nutrition therapy*, a term used to describe guidance and intervention by a dieticians.

Table 2.11 Nutrient composition of the therapeutic lifestyle changes (TLC) diet[a]

Nutrient	Recommended intake
Saturated fat[a]	Less than 7% of total calories
Polyunsaturated fat	Up to 10% of total calories
Monounsaturated fat	Up to 20% of total calories
Total fat	25%–35% of total calories
Carbohydrate[b]	50%–60% of total calories
Fiber	20–30 g/day
Protein	~15% of total calories
Cholesterol	Less than 200 mg/day
Total calories (energy)[c]	Maintain desirable body weight/prevent weight gain

[a]*trans* fatty acids are another LDL-raising fat that should be kept at a low intake.
[b]Carbohydrate should be derived predominantly from foods rich in complex carbohydrates including grains, especially whole grains, fruits, and vegetables.
[c]Daily energy expenditure should include at least moderate physical activity (contributing ~200 Kcal/day).
Source: Adapted with permission from National Cholesterol Education Program (NCEP) Expert Panel on Detection, Evaluation, and Treatment of High Blood Cholesterol in Adults (Adult Treatment Panel III). Third Report of the National Cholesterol Education Program (NCEP) Expert Panel on Detection, Evaluation, and Treatment of High Blood Cholesterol in Adults (Adult Treatment Panel III) final report. Circulation 2002;106:3143–3421.

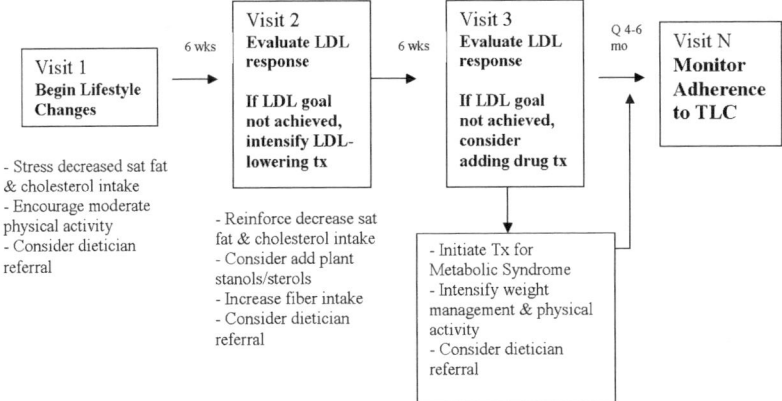

Fig. 2.1 A model of steps in therapeutic lifestyle changes (*TLC*). *LDL*, low density lipoprotein; *sat*, saturated; Tx, treatment. [Adapted with permission from National Cholesterol Education Program (NCEP) Expert Panel on Detection, Evaluation, and Treatment of High Blood Cholesterol in Adults (Adult Treatment Panel III). Third Report of the National Cholesterol Education Program (NCEP) Expert Panel on Detection, Evaluation, and Treatment of High Blood Cholesterol in Adults (Adult Treatment Panel III) final report. Circulation 2002;106:3143–3421.]

Drug Therapy to Achieve LDL Cholesterol Goals

Although the evidence presented in ATP III clearly advocated that emphasis should be placed on the use of TLC in all patients with elevated CHD risk, it also recognized that some of these patients would require LDL-lowering drugs to reach optimal LDL cholesterol levels. As previously shown in Fig. 2.1, if LDL goals have not been met within 3 months of TLC initiation, consideration should be given to adding lipid-lowering medications. This report also recognized the need for simultaneous initiation of TLC and LDL-lowering therapy for patients with severe hyperlipidemia and for those patients with CHD or CHD risk equivalent in which dietary therapy would be unlikely to achieve suggested LDL goals. Figure 2.2 depicts the panel's proposed drug therapy progression model.

ATP III formally established HMG CoA reductase inhibitors (statins) as first-line medications for LDL cholesterol lowering. In addition, this panel recommended consideration of bile acid sequestrants for the following uses: (1) for patients with moderate elevations in LDL cholesterol; (2) for younger patients with elevated LDL cholesterol; (3) for women considering pregnancy; (4) for patients needing only modest LDL cholesterol reductions to reach goal LDL levels; and (5) for combination therapy with statins in patients with significantly elevated LDL cholesterol levels.

ATP III also confirmed evidence that nicotinic acid reduced triglyceride-rich lipoprotein remnants, raised HDL cholesterol, increased the size of LDL particles, and caused moderate reductions in LDL cholesterol levels. The 2002 report also recognized evidence that nicotinic acid produced moderate decreases in CHD risk alone or in combination with other lipid-lowering medications. Additionally, the panel recommended that nicotinic acid be considered for higher-risk patients with atherogenic dyslipidemia who do not have significantly increased LDL cholesterol levels as well as recommending its use in combination with other lipid-lowering medications in higher-risk patients with atherogenic dyslipidemia and high LDL cholesterol levels.

Fibrate medications were reported to be successful in modifying atherogenic dyslipidemia, with particular effect on serum triglyceride levels as well as some

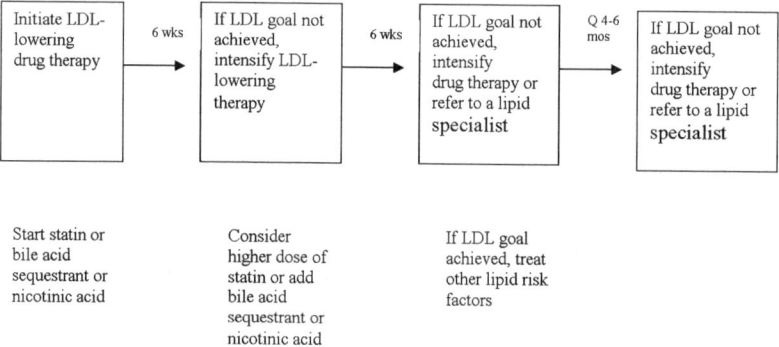

Fig. 2.2 Progression of drug therapy. [Adapted with permission from National Cholesterol Education Program (NCEP) Expert Panel on Detection, Evaluation, and Treatment of High Blood Cholesterol in Adults (Adult Treatment Panel III). Third Report of the National Cholesterol Education Program (NCEP) Expert Panel on Detection, Evaluation, and Treatment of High Blood Cholesterol in Adults (Adult Treatment Panel III) final report. Circulation 2002;106:3143–3421.]

lowering of LDL cholesterol levels. In addition, ATP III noted evidence that fibrate therapy reduced the risk for CHD as well as stroke risk in secondary prevention. Based on this information, the report endorsed fibrates for the treatment of patients with high triglycerides to reduce the risk of pancreatitis and for patients with elevated beta very low density lipoprotein (VLDL).

Drug Therapy for Secondary Prevention in Hospitalized Patients

ATP III established the LDL cholesterol goal of less than 100 for patients with known CHD and CHD risk equivalents. The report recommended that all patients admitted to the hospital for a major coronary event have a LDL cholesterol measured within 24 h of admission or at least before discharge. Furthermore, it recommended basing treatment decisions upon the results, and, if LDL cholesterol was 130 mg/dl or higher, the report recommended initiation of lipid-lowering medications, with clinical judgment being used when the values fell between 100 and 129 mg/dl. The report recognized two substantial benefits from starting LDL-lowering medications in hospitalized patients with CHD-related illness and a LDL cholesterol greater than 100 mg/dl. The benefits were high patient motivation and closure of the "treatment gap" for those with poor compliance with treatment.

LDL-Lowering Drug Therapy for Primary Prevention

Figure 2.2 also applies when lipid-lowering medications are being considered for primary prevention of CHD. Table 2.12 outlines the ATP III recommended

Table 2.12 Drug therapy consideration and goals of therapy for primary prevention

Risk category	Ten-year risk for CHD	Level at which to consider drug therapy	Primary goal of therapy
Multiple (2+) risk factors	More than 20% (includes all CHD risk equivalents	More than 100 mg/dl[a]	Less than 100 mg/dl
	10%–20%	$\geq$130 mg/dl[b]	<130 mg/dl
	<10%	$\geq$160 mg/dl	<130 mg/dl
0–1 risk factor	<10%	$\geq$190 mg/dl[c]	<160 mg/dl

[a]When LDL cholesterol is $\geq$130 mg/dl, a cholesterol-lowering drug can be started concomitantly with TLC. If baseline LDL is 100–129 mg/dl, TLC should be started immediately. Concomitant use of drugs is optional; several options for drug therapy are available.
[b]When LDL is in the range of 130–159 mg/dl, drug therapy can be used if necessary to reach the LDL-cholesterol goal of <130 mg/dl, after an adequate trial of TLC.
[c]When LDL cholesterol is in the range of 160–189 mg/dl, use of cholesterol-lowering medications is optional, depending on response to TLC diet.
Source. Adapted with permission from National Cholesterol Education Program (NCEP) Expert Panel on Detection, Evaluation, and Treatment of High Blood Cholesterol in Adults (Adult Treatment Panel III). Third Report of the National Cholesterol Education Program (NCEP) Expert Panel on Detection, Evaluation, and Treatment of High Blood Cholesterol in Adults (Adult Treatment Panel III) final report. Circulation 2002;106:3143–3421.

approach to the use of drug therapy for primary prevention of CHD as it relates to differing risk categories.

ATP III stresses that it is vital to emphasize TLC to all patients with lipid disorders, and the highest priority is to reduce LDL cholesterol below goals set by the report. The report recommended starting medication at moderate dosages and recognized that high-dose ranges will rarely be necessary to reach goal if TLC is emphasized and maintained.

Metabolic Syndrome as a Secondary Target of Therapy

ATP III reported the mounting evidence that CHD risk could be reduced by tempering other risk factors. The panel stressed that the goal of metabolic syndrome management was to reduce obesity and physical inactivity while simultaneously treating associated lipid and nonlipid risk factors.

Management of Underlying Causes of the Metabolic Syndrome

Weight reduction and increased physical activity are emphasized as primary targets of therapy for metabolic syndrome treatment once LDL cholesterol control is obtained. The report references the NHLBI Obesity Education Initiative for recommended approaches to weight loss intervention [7]. The report also recognized the role of physical activity in reducing VLDL and, in some cases, LDL, while simultaneously elevating HDL levels. Furthermore, it noted that physical activity lowered blood pressure, reduced insulin resistance, and had beneficial effects on cardiovascular function. The report cites the U.S. Surgeon General's Report on Physical Activity as the evidence base for this recommendation [8]. Finally, the report acknowledged that the treatment of hypertension, elevated triglycerides, and low HDL in addition to the use of aspirin in patients with CHD will further reduce CHD risk in patients with metabolic syndrome.

Special Issues

Management of Specific Dyslipidemias

The importance of detecting genetic forms of lipid disorders in patients with LDL cholesterol levels of 190 mg/dl or more was emphasized. In addition to advocating for use of combination drug therapy to achieve recommended lipid goals when necessary, the report also recommended cholesterol testing in young adults to prevent early CHD in patients with genetic lipid disorders. The three most common genetic lipid disorders are familial hypercholesterolemia (FH), familial defective apolipoprotein B-100 (FDB), and polygenic hypercholesterolemia.

Heterozygous FH is an autosomal-dominant disorder with a prevalence of 1 in 500 people [9]. Hypercholesterolemia is generally detectable shortly after birth, with total cholesterol levels rising to 350–500 mg/dl. Tendon xanthomas are typical, most commonly occur on the Achilles tendon or the extensor tendon of the hands, and may require two- or three-drug therapy to reach goals.

Homozygous FH occurs in approximately 1 in 1 million people [9]. This disorder is characterized by defective LDL receptors, total cholesterol levels of 700–1200 mg/day, early cutaneous xanthomas, and late tendon and tuberous xanthomas. As a result of the defective LDL receptors, this disorder is recalcitrant to diet changes and drug therapy. ATP III reported that plasmaphoresis was the therapeutic mode of choice.

FDB is another autosomal-dominant disorder resulting from a nucleotide mutation in apolipoprotein B. This mutation reduces affinity of the LDL particle for the LDL receptor, causing elevated LDL levels. The prevalence of FDB is about 1 in 700–1000 people [10]. Diagnosis requires molecular screening in specialized laboratories, and treatment is similar to that for FH.

Polygenic hypercholesterolemia patients have LDL levels of 190 mg/dl or more, and the total cholesterol elevation is usually less than that of patients with heterozygous FH. Furthermore, tendon xanthomas are not observed. Therapy is essentially the same as for patients with FH with drug combination therapy.

Elevated Triglycerides

Elevated triglycerides were identified in the report as an independent CHD risk factor based on prior meta-analyses. It reported that higher than normal triglycerides were seen in patients with obesity, overweight, physical inactivity, cigarette smoking, alcohol excess, high-carbohydrate diets, certain disease states (type 2 DM, chronic renal failure, nephritic syndrome), and individual drugs (corticosteroids, estrogens, retinoids, beta-blockers, antiretrovirals), as well as some genetic maladies (familial combined hyperlipidemia, familial hypertriglyceridemia, and familial dysbetalipoproteinemia). The report also adopted the triglyceride classification noted below:

> Normal: less than 150 mg/dl
> Borderline: 150–199 mg/dl
> High: 200–499 mg/dl
> Very high: 500 mg/dl or more

Once triglycerides were identified as an independent risk factor, this prompted research to find the offending triglyceride-rich lipoproteins. It was found that partially degraded VLDL particles called remnant lipoproteins are atherogenic. Clinically, VLDL cholesterol is the most accessible measure of these remnant lipoproteins, and, as such, it can be a target of therapy. ATP III recognized the LDL + VLDL aggregate (coined as *non-HDL cholesterol*) as a secondary objective of

Table 2.13 Comparison of LDL cholesterol and non-HDL cholesterol (C) goals for three risk categories

Risk category	LDL goal (mg/dl)	Non-HDL-C goal (mg/dl)
CHD and CHD Risk equivalents (10-year risk for CHD >20%)	<100	<130
Multiple (2+) risk factors + 10-year risk ≤20%	<130	<160
0–1 risk factor	<160	<190

Source: Adapted with permission from National Cholesterol Education Program (NCEP) Expert Panel on Detection, Evaluation, and Treatment of High Blood Cholesterol in Adults (Adult Treatment Panel III). Third Report of the National Cholesterol Education Program (NCEP) Expert Panel on Detection, Evaluation, and Treatment of High Blood Cholesterol in Adults (Adult Treatment Panel III) final report. Circulation 2002;106:3143–3421.

therapy in patients with elevated triglycerides (200 mg/dl or more). The goal for patients with elevated triglycerides is a non-HDL cholesterol 30 mg/dl higher than the LDL goal (Table 2.13).

The report further conveyed that the therapeutic approach to patients with high triglycerides depended on the cause and degree of the increased levels. Weight reduction and increased physical activity were recommended for those patients with borderline high triglycerides (150–199 mg/dl). In patients with high triglycerides (200–499 mg/dl), the report recommends that the secondary target of lowering non-HDL cholesterol be added. In high-risk patients, pharmacotherapy can be added to attain the non-HDL cholesterol goal. ATP III suggested two drug therapy schemes to use in such cases: (1) intensifying LDL-lowering drug therapy or (2) adding nicotinic acid or fibrates.

Preventing acute pancreatitis by lowering triglycerides is the initial primary goal of therapy in those patients with very high (500 mg/dl or more) triglyceride levels, and, once the level is below 500 mg/dl, attention can turn toward lowering LDL levels to decrease CHD risk.

HDL Cholesterol

HDL levels were also noted to be a stand-alone predictor of CHD in this report, and their relationship to triglyceride levels was identified. The report redefined low HDL cholesterol as less than 40 mg/dl in men and less than 50 mg/dl in premenopausal women, which was a significant change from the ATP II level of less than 35 mg/dl. Although identified as multifactorial, most causes of low-HDL cholesterol were identified as being associated with insulin resistance (type 2 diabetes, physical inactivity, obesity, and elevated triglycerides), smoking, high carbohydrate intake, and medications (beta-blockers, anabolic steroids, progestational agents). This report does not recommend a specific HDL goal, but clinical trials cited suggested that elevating HDL would reduce CHD risk. It does, however, recommend a sequence for the clinical management of low HDL levels. Once LDL goals are achieved, HDL can be raised by (1) shifting emphasis to weight reduction and increased physical activity in the presence of metabolic syndrome; (2) achieving non-HDL cholesterol goals when high triglyceride levels exist; and (3) considering HDL-raising medications (nicotinic acid or fibrates) if triglycerides are less than 200 mg/dl.

Diabetes Mellitus

Diabetes was recognized by ATP III as a CHD risk equivalent. The report points to an LDL goal of less than 100 mg/dl as the primary target of therapy despite the common presence of elevated triglycerides and low HDL in these patients. It stressed that if LDL cholesterol was 130 mg/dl or higher, most diabetics would require drug therapy *and* TLC to achieve goal LDL levels. Additionally, it stated that if LDL fell between 100 and 129 mg/dl, diabetics had multiple therapeutic options, including (1) increasing the intensity of LDL-lowering medication therapy; (2) adding fibrates or nicotinic acid to modify atherogenic dyslipidemia; and (3) increased control of other modifiable risk factors including hyperglycemia, hypertension, insulin resistance, and cigarette smoking. When diabetics have triglyceride levels of 200 mg/dl or more, the report recommends that non-HDL cholesterol be the secondary therapeutic objective. Fibrates and low-dose nicotinic acid may lead to a non-HDL level less than 130 mg/dl.

Special Considerations for Different Population Groups

In recognition of the fact that middle-aged men (35–65 years of age) carry a relatively high CHD risk and that they are predisposed to abdominal obesity and metabolic syndrome, ATP III recommended intensive LDL-lowering therapy at the time of identification. The report also recognized that women begin development of CHD some 10–15 years later than men. In those women with premature onset of CHD (less than 65 years old), most have multiple risk factors and metabolic syndrome.

In relation to older patients (men older than 65 years and women older than 75 years), this review cited that these patients experience the most new CHD events and coronary-related deaths [11]. As such, ATP III recognized that no rigid age restrictions are necessary when considering LDL-lowering therapy for older patients with CHD. The report calls for TLC as the first-line therapy in these patients and LDL-lowering medications when high CHD risk is present as a consequence of multiple risk factors or advanced subclinical atherosclerosis. ATP III also recommended using number-needed-to-treat (NNT) data when considering lipid-lowering medications (Table 2.14).

In relation to younger patients (men 20–35 years of age; women 20–45 years of age), the report noted they experience rare CHD events unless severe risk factors

Table 2.14 Number needed to treat (NNT) with statin therapy for 15 years to prevent CHD events by age 80 starting at age 65[a]

10-year risk for CHD	CHD death	NNT to prevent CHD events (15 years of drug therapy) Hard CHD[b]	Total CHD[c]
10%	42	21	10
20%	20	10	5
30%	13	7	3
40%	10	5	1–2

[a]The results in this table assume that statin therapy reduces relative risk for all CHD events by one-third.

[b]Hard CHD included MI + CHD death.

[c]Total CHD includes MI, CHD death, unstable angina, and coronary procedures (angioplasty, CABG).

Source: Adapted with permission from National Cholesterol Education Program (NCEP) Expert Panel on Detection, Evaluation, and Treatment of High Blood Cholesterol in Adults (Adult Treatment Panel III). Third Report of the National Cholesterol Education Program (NCEP) Expert Panel on Detection, Evaluation, and Treatment of High Blood Cholesterol in Adults (Adult Treatment Panel III) final report. Circulation 2002;106:3143–3421.

are present (diabetes, heavy smoking, or familial hypercholesterolemia). ATP III recognized that an increase in serum cholesterol levels in young adulthood does increase risk for premature CHD in middle age. Early detection and intervention when LDL cholesterol is elevated in young adults are endorsed. Delayed-onset or true CHD prevention can be afforded with life habit changes when LDL cholesterol is 130 mg/dl or higher. ATP III advocates consideration of lipid-lowering medications in young men who smoke and have high cholesterol levels (160–189 mg/dl) as well as young men who have very high LDL cholesterol levels (190 mg/dl or higher) and zero or one risk factor.

ATP III recognized that African Americans have the highest overall CHD mortality rate and the highest out-of-hospital death rates from CHD when compared to other ethnic groups in the United States. Hypertension, left ventricular hypertrophy, diabetes, cigarette smoking, physical activity, obesity, and other risk factors were recognized as more prevalent when comparing African Americans to white Americans. Modifications of general ATP III evidence-based lipid management recommendations were not warranted by the differences in ethnic group. However, ATP III advocated that particular attention be given to the detection and control of hypertension in African Americans.

ATP III also acknowledged mild baseline risk differences between white Americans and other ethnic groups (Hispanics, Native Americans, Asian, Pacific Islanders, and South Asians), but it did not recommend using separate guidelines for these populations. Special populations are discussed further in Chapter 7.

Adherence to LDL-Lowering Therapy

ATP III recommended the use of multidisciplinary methods to target the patients, the providers, and the healthcare delivery systems to accomplish the goals outlined

Table 2.15 Interventions to improve adherence

Focus on the patient:

- Simplify medication regimens
- Provide explicit patient instructions and use good counseling techniques to teach the patient how to follow the prescribed treatment
- Encourage the use of prompts to help patients remember treatment regimens
- Use systems to reinforce adherence and maintain contact with the patient
- Encourage the support of family and friends
- Reinforce and reward adherence
- Increase visits for patients unable to achieve treatment goal
- Increase the convenience and access to care
- Involve patients in their care through self-monitoring

Focus on the physician and medical office:

- Teach physicians to implement lipid treatment guidelines
- Use reminders to prompt physicians to attend to lipid management
- Identify a patient advocate in the office to help deliver or prompt care
- Use patients to prompt preventive care
- Develop a standardized treatment plan to structure care
- Use feedback from past performance to foster change in future care
- Remind patients of appointments and follow-up missed appointments

Focus on health delivery system:

- Provide lipid management through a lipid clinic
- Utilize case management by nurses
- Deploy telemedicine
- Utilize the collaborative care of pharmacists
- Execute critical care pathways in hospitals

Source: Adapted with permission from National Cholesterol Education Program (NCEP) Expert Panel on Detection, Evaluation, and Treatment of High Blood Cholesterol in Adults (Adult Treatment Panel III). Third Report of the National Cholesterol Education Program (NCEP) Expert Panel on Detection, Evaluation, and Treatment of High Blood Cholesterol in Adults (Adult Treatment Panel III) final report. Circulation 2002;106:3143–3421.

for primary and secondary prevention of CHD (Table 2.15). Table 2.16 provides a simple method for clinicians to use to improve adherence to LDL-lowering regimens.

The 2004 NCEP ATP-III Update

Subsequent to the ATP III Report, in the July 13, 2004 issue of *Circulation*, the NCEP made additional recommendations and modifications based on new data from five major clinical trials [2]. The studies reviewed in this publication were (1) Heart Protection Study (HPS); (2) Prospective Study of Pravastatin in the Elderly at Risk (PROSPER); (3) Antihypertensive and Lipid-Lowering Treatment to Prevent Heart Attack Trial—Lipid-Lowering Trial (ALLHAT-LLT); (4) Scandinavian Cardiac Outcomes Trial—Lipid-Lowering Arm (ASCOT-LLA); and (5) Pravastatin or Atorvastatin Evaluation and Infection Therapy—Thrombolysis in

Table 2.16 The Clinician's Abridged Pocket Guide to Enhancing Adherence

- Keep the regimen as simple as possible
- Give the patient clear instructions
- Discuss adherence for at least a few seconds at each visit
- Concentrate on those who do not reach treatment goals
- Always call patients who miss visit appointments
- Use two or more strategies for those who miss treatment goals

Source: Adapted with permission from National Cholesterol Education Program (NCEP) Expert Panel on Detection, Evaluation, and Treatment of High Blood Cholesterol in Adults (Adult Treatment Panel III). Third Report of the National Cholesterol Education Program (NCEP) Expert Panel on Detection, Evaluation, and Treatment of High Blood Cholesterol in Adults (Adult Treatment Panel III) final report. Circulation 2002;106:3143–3421.

Myocardial Infarction 22 (PROVE IT-TIMI 22). Each of these studies was reviewed in Chapter 1.

Although therapeutic lifestyle changes (TLC) remained a cornerstone of treatment in all risk groups, these new studies both supported and expanded the recommendations that ATP-III was able to make regarding high-risk, moderate-risk, diabetic, relatively low LDL cholesterol (LDL-C), and elderly patients. The proposed modifications to ATP III recommendations based on this new clinical evidence included the following:

1. Although the recommended LDL-C goal for high-risk patients remained at less than 100 mg/dl, a target of less than 70 mg/dl was noted to be a reasonable therapeutic goal for those at very high risk:

    a. If the baseline LDL-C level is 130 mg/dl or greater, simultaneous initiation of pharmacotherapy and TLC is recommended.

    b. If the LDL-C is 100 to 129 mg/dl, both pharmacotherapy and TLC are indicated.

    c. High-risk patients with elevated triglycerides (200 mg/dl or greater) or low HDL-C levels might require the addition of a fibrate or nicotinic acid to LDL-lowering therapy.

    d. If an LDL-C lowering drug was used for a high-risk patient, then a reduction of LDL-C levels of at least 30% to 40% should be achieved, regardless of ATP III goals.

2. Although the LDL-C goal for moderately high risk (Framingham 10-year risk of 10%–20%) patients remained less than 130 mg/dl, a goal of less than 100 mg/dl had strong clinical evidence of risk reduction and was deemed to be a valid therapeutic option:

    a. If the LDL-C remained at 130 mg/dl or greater after TLC, strong consideration should be given to starting an LDL-lowering drug.

    b. If an LDL-lowering drug was used in a moderately high risk patient, then a reduction of LDL-C levels of at least 30% to 40% should be achieved, regardless of ATP III goals.

Table 2.17 LDL cholesterol goals and cutpoints for therapeutic lifestyle changes (TLC) and drug therapy in different risk categories: 2004 update

Risk category	LDL goal	LDL level at which to initiate TLC	LDL level at which to consider drug therapy
High risk			
CHD or CHD Equivalents or (10-year risk >20%)	<100 mg/dl Optional goal <70 mg/dl[a]	≥100 mg/dl	≥100 mg/dl (<100 mg/dl; consider drugs)
Moderately high risk			
2+ risk factors (10-year risk 10%–20%)	<130 mg/dl Optional goal <100 mg/dl	≥130 mg/dl	≥130 mg/dl (100–129 mg/dl; consider drug options)
Moderate risk			
2+ risk factors (10-year risk <10%)	<130 mg/dl	≥130 mg/dl	≥160 mg/dl
Low risk			
0–1 risk factors	<160 mg/dl	≥160 mg/dl	≥190 mg/dl (160–190 mg/dl; consider drugs)

[a]Current evidence for high-risk patients favors the optional goal of less than 70 mg/dl.
Source: Adapted with permission from Grundy SM, Cleeman JI, Merz CNB, et al. Implications of recent clinical trials for the National Cholesterol Education Program Adult Treatment Panel III Guidelines. Circulation 2004;110:227–239.

No recommendations for modification of goals for lower-risk patients were made in the update. Table 2.17 provides a summary of goals and cutpoints for TLC and drug therapy in different risk categories.

References

1. National Cholesterol Education Program (NCEP) Expert Panel on Detection, Evaluation, and Treatment of High Blood Cholesterol in Adults (Adult Treatment Panel III). Third Report of the National Cholesterol Education Program (NCEP) Expert Panel on Detection, Evaluation, and Treatment of High Blood Cholesterol in Adults (Adult Treatment Panel III) final report. Circulation 2002;106:3143–3421.
2. Grundy SM, Cleeman JI, Merz CN, Brewer HB Jr, Clark LT, Hunninghake DB, Pasternak RC, Smith SC Jr, Stone NJ. Implications of recent clinical trials for the National Cholesterol Education Program Adult Treatment Panel III guidelines. Circulation 2004;110: 227–239.
3. National Cholesterol Education Program (NCEP) Expert Panel on Detection, Evaluation, and Treatment of High Blood Cholesterol in Adults (Adult Treatment Panel III). Third Report of the National Cholesterol Education Program (NCEP) Expert Panel on Detection, Evaluation, and Treatment of High Blood Cholesterol in Adults (Adult Treatment Panel III) final report. Circulation 2002;106:12.
4. Report of the National Cholesterol Education Program Expert Panel on Detection, Evaluation, and Treatment of High Blood Cholesterol in Adults: the Expert Panel. Arch Intern Med 1988:36–69.

5. National Cholesterol Education Program. Second report of the expert panel on detection, evaluation, and treatment of high blood cholesterol in adults (Adult Treatment Panel II). Circulation 1994;89:1333–1445.
6. National Cholesterol Education Program (NCEP) Expert Panel on Detection, Evaluation, and Treatment of High Blood Cholesterol in Adults (Adult Treatment Panel III). Third Report of the National Cholesterol Education Program (NCEP) Expert Panel on Detection, Evaluation, and Treatment of High Blood Cholesterol in Adults (Adult Treatment Panel III) final report. Circulation 2002;106:62.
7. National Institutes of Health. Clinical guidelines on the identification, evaluation and treatment of overweight and obesity in adults: the evidence report. Obes Res 1998;6(suppl 2): 51S–209S.
8. U.S. Department of Health and Human Services. Physical activity and health: a Report of the Surgeon General. Atlanta, GA: U.S. Department of Health and Human Services, Centers for Disease Control and Prevention, National Center for Chronic Disease Prevention and Health Promotion, 1996.
9. Goldstein JI, Brown MS. Familial hypercholesterolemia. In: Scriver CR., Beaudet AL, Sty WS, et al (eds) The metabolic basis of inherited disease. New York: McGraw-Hill, 1995:1981–2030.
10. Innerarity TL, Mahley RW, Weisgraber KH, et al. Familial defective apolipoprotein B-100: a mutation of apolipoprotein B that causes hypercholesterolemia. J Lipid Res 1990;31: 1337–1349.
11. National Center for Health Statistics. Fulwood R, Kalsbeek W, Rifkind B, et al. Total serum cholesterol levels of adults 20–74 years of age: U.S., 1976–80. Vital and Health Statistics, series 11. No. 236. DHHS Publ. No. (PHS) 86-1686. Washington, DC: National Center for Health Statistics, Public Health Service, U.S. Government Printing Office, May 1986.

Suggested Key Readings

Grundy SM, Cleeman JI, Merz CN, Brewer HB Jr, Clark LT, Hunninghake DB, Pasternak RC, Smith SC Jr, Stone NJ. Implications of recent clinical trials for the National Cholesterol Education Program Adult Treatment Panel III guidelines. Circulation 2004;110: 227–239.
National Cholesterol Education Program (NCEP) Expert Panel on Detection, Evaluation, and Treatment of High Blood Cholesterol in Adults (Adult Treatment Panel III). Third Report of the National Cholesterol Education Program (NCEP) Expert Panel on Detection, Evaluation, and Treatment of High Blood Cholesterol in Adults (Adult Treatment Panel III) final report. Circulation 2002;106:3143–3421.

Chapter 3
Dietary Interventions

Christopher W. Walker

Introduction

Obesity has reached epidemic proportions in the United States, with data from the 1999–2002 National Health and Nutrition Examination Survey showing that approximately 65% of adults are either overweight or obese [1]. Obesity, especially abdominal adiposity, is a major risk factor for a number of known cardiovascular risk factors including dyslipidemia, hypertension, and diabetes mellitus [2]. Furthermore, low density lipoprotein (LDL) cholesterol levels have been shown to rise in response to increased intake of dietary cholesterol and saturated fats. Therefore, dietary counseling has become a key treatment strategy for healthcare providers treating their patients with dyslipidemia. The 2004 update to the National Cholesterol Education Program (NCEP) guidelines can necessitate more than 50% reductions in LDL in some patients. This level of reduction is difficult to achieve with medication or dietary intervention alone. Last, several dietary interventions have been shown to lower cardiovascular risk independent of lipid lowering.

The present-day patient is faced with a confusing myriad of dietary choices in the print media and on the Internet [3]. Patients who manifest obesity and hyperlipidemia will be best served by a diet that reduces the maximum number of risk factors for coronary artery disease and offers sustainable weight loss or maintenance.

The dietary approaches and plans discussed in this chapter fall into two categories: those that were developed and marketed for the goal of weight loss, and those which were developed to ameliorate very specific coronary risk factors. Despite the developer's intent, most of these nutritional strategies can have an effect on both these endpoints. A primary care healthcare provider must be educated about these diets so that sound advice can be delivered to patients hoping to achieve either

C.W. Walker
Associate Program Director, David Grant Family Medicine Residency Program, Department of Family Medicine, University of California at Davis Affiliate Program/David Grant Medical Center, Travis Air Force Base, CA

B.V. Reamy (ed.), *Hyperlipidemia Management for Primary Care*,
DOI: 10.1007/978-0-387-76606-5_3, © Springer Science+Business Media, LLC 2008

Table 3.1 Dietary interventions and lipid parameters

Diet	LDL	HDL	Triglycerides	Cardiovascular event reduction	Level of evidence[a]
NCEP Step 1 [47–60,62]	Decrease	No change	No change	No event data	B
NCEP Step 2 [47–60,62]	Decrease	Decrease	No change	No event data	B
Therapeutic lifestyle changes (TLC) [47]	Decrease	Decrease	No change	No event data	A
Very low fat (less than 10%) [13,17,19–21]	Decrease	Decrease	Decrease	Decrease	B
Low carbohydrate [4–9,12]	No change	Increase	Decrease	No event data	B
Moderate carbohydrate/low glycemic index [23,24,25,26,28]	No change	No change	No change	No event data	B
Mediterranean diet [29–40,42–46, 68,69]	Decrease/no change	Increase	Decrease	Decrease	A

[a]A, recommendation based on consistent and good-quality patient-oriented evidence; B, recommendation based on inconsistent or limited quality patient-oriented evidence; C, recommendation based on consensus, usual practice, opinion, disease-oriented evidence, and case series for studies of diagnosis, treatment, prevention, or screening.

weight loss or the amelioration of specific coronary risk factors. Table 3.1 is a summary of the evidence on the effects of dietary interventions on lipid values.

Low-Carbohydrate Diets

Atkins Diet

First published by Dr. Robert Atkins in 1972, the Atkins Diet is the most popular and best studied of the low-carbohydrate, non-calorie-restricted diets [4]. It is also the diet that is most commonly modeled in studies of low-carbohydrate diets. The diet consists of a four-phase plan with an *induction period* marked by severe limitation of dietary carbohydrates (less than 20 g/day). The following phases also restrict carbohydrates, with the addition of 5–10 net carbohydrates/grams per week, utilizing weight change or lack of urine ketosis as a marker for overindulgence of carbohydrates. Dieters who desire further weight loss are encouraged to move back to earlier stages and increase carbohydrate restriction. Of note, this diet does *not* have any caloric restrictions or portion restrictions. Earlier versions of the diet encouraged liberal intake of foods high in saturated fat. The most recent iteration of this diet does incorporate recommendations for increased fat intake from healthier sources such as fish and olive oil.

The largest concerns regarding this diet have focused on a potential increase in dietary cholesterol and saturated fat with a concomitant reduction of fruits and vegetables with the imposition of severe carbohydrate restriction. Critics have surmised that these restrictions may lead to an increase in cardiovascular and cancer risks. Until recently, these concerns had not been addressed in the scientific literature.

Until 2003, there were very few randomized controlled studies evaluating the effectiveness of high-fat/low-carbohydrate diets in causing and maintaining weight loss. Many of the studies that have been published since that time have included lipid levels as primary or secondary endpoints. All the studies involved were confounded by poor compliance, with most reporting attrition rates of 20% to 40% in the treatment and control groups. It should be noted that most weight loss studies involving other diets and community-based (nonhospitalized) patients have similar high attrition rates. Another limitation of these trials was the short study length, with none lasting for longer than 1 year.

Cardiovascular Risk Factor Endpoints

LDL Cholesterol

Yancy et al. studied 120 *hyperlipidemic, obese* patients randomized to a low-carbohydrate diet or a low-fat diet. These dieters were studied for 6 months. At the end of this time period, there was no significant difference between their LDL levels despite the fact that the low-carbohydrate dieters lost significantly more weight [5]. Two of the patients in the low-carbohydrate group withdrew from the study because of rapid increase in LDL levels. However, the overall results showed *no beneficial or adverse affects* of this diet on this important marker for cardiovascular disease.

Foster et al. studied the effect of a low-carbohydrate diet versus a low-fat, calorie-restricted diet on 63 obese men and women for 1 year, observing weight loss, lipids, diastolic blood pressure, and insulin response to glucose load [6]. At the end of 6 months, the intervention group saw the same weight loss differential as the aforementioned study; however, there was no significant difference in weight at 1 year. Of the 59% of dieters who completed the study, there was a trend toward a lower LDL in the low-fat dieters; this trend did not meet statistical significance. Again, there was no significant change in LDL levels in the low-carbohydrate dieters.

Studies performed in higher-risk patients have shown similar results with regard to LDL levels. Samaha et al. studied 132 severely obese patients with a mean body mass index of 43 who were randomized to a low-carbohydrate or low-fat diet for 6 months. Moreover, 39% of these patients had *diabetes*, and 43% of those without diabetes met the criteria for the *metabolic syndrome*. Despite greater weight loss in the low-carbohydrate dieters, there was no significant change in LDL levels [7]. The same researchers reported lipoprotein subfractions in this group of patients in a later paper [8]. They found that the low-carbohydrate diet resulted in a greater decrease in large very low density lipoprotein (VLDL) concentrations; however, these patients also developed higher levels of circulating chylomicrons while in a fasting state. Decreased large VLDL concentrations are thought to decrease cardiovascular risk, whereas circulating chylomicrons may lead to the development of unstable arterial plaques through increased macrophage uptake of fat precursors and plaque inflammation. Again, no significant difference was found between dietary groups in LDL subfraction concentrations. The clinical implications of this study are unclear.

There is a paucity of research in the pediatric population with a low-carbohydrate diet; however, Sondike et al. studied the effect of low-carbohydrate diets on cardiovascular risk factors in overweight adolescent patients over a 12-week period [9]. Although the low-carbohydrate diet resulted in significantly more weight loss, it neither worsened nor improved LDL levels. The patients on the low-fat diet did, however, show an improvement in their LDL levels, with a drop of approximately 20%.

Although there are a few studies of shorter duration (less than 12 weeks) that show increasing LDL levels with a low-carbohydrate diet, all the larger, randomized studies demonstrated no significant change from baseline despite greater weight loss at 6 months and equivalent weight loss at 1 year.

> **Conclusion:** Of the multiple randomized trials that evaluated LDL cholesterol as an endpoint in low-carbohydrate diets, none showed significant improvements compared to control groups of low-fat dieters.

HDL Cholesterol/Triglycerides

Decreased high density lipoprotein (HDL) cholesterol is a known independent risk factor for coronary artery disease. The link to triglyceride elevation and coronary disease is less clear because elevated triglycerides are frequently associated with a decreased HDL level as well as diabetes and the metabolic syndrome [10,11].

All the aforementioned studies evaluated triglycerides and HDL cholesterol (HDL-C) levels in low-carbohydrate diets in comparison to low-fat diets. The results were mixed. Samaha et al. demonstrated that a low-carbohydrate diet did not significantly change HDL-C, but decreased triglyceride levels by 20% over 6 months in severely obese patients, with a large portion of participants who were also diabetic; this is in contrast to a 4% triglyceride decrease in the same dieters on a low-fat diet [7]. These results were replicated by Meckling et al. in otherwise healthy overweight men and women, although both low-fat and low-carbohydrate dieters showed a similar decrease in triglycerides [12]. In the longest study of low-carbohydrate diets and cardiac risk factors, Foster et al. showed that there was a significant reduction in triglycerides (TG) and elevation in HDL that persisted at 12 months in the low-carbohydrate group [6]. The low-carbohydrate dieters HDL and TG levels were also significantly better than their low-fat counterparts. In fact, the mean reduction in TG of 28% in the low-carbohydrate group matches the decrease that can be expected with fibrate drugs or niacin.

Researchers are hesitant to attach clinical significance to these profile improvements. HDL elevation by increased saturated fat intake has not been studied exclusively with clinical outcomes as an endpoint. Proponents of very low fat diets argue that increasing HDL by increasing saturated fat may actually worsen heart disease risk by other inflammatory mechanisms that are not reflected by the serum lipid levels. This is an area that deserves further, long-term study [13].

> **Conclusion:** Low-carbohydrate diets appear to decrease triglycerides and raise HDL cholesterol levels. The clinical impact of these changes is unknown.

Meta-Analyses of Low-Carbohydrate Diets

A large meta-analysis of the randomized controlled trials of low-carbohydrate diets was undertaken by Nordmann et al. in 2006. The paper limited its scope to studies comparing non-energy-restricted, low-carbohydrate diets to energy-restricted low-fat diets. Trials included participants with a body mass index (BMI) greater than 25 with a follow-up duration of at least 6 months. These criteria allowed for the analysis of six trials with a total of 447 participants. The results of the pooled data analysis confirmed what many of the larger individual trials had shown. In short, low-carbohydrate diets are more effective for short-term weight loss (6 months or less) but are equal to low-fat diets at 1 year. There were no differences in blood pressure parameters after 1 year. There was a nonsignificant trend toward higher total cholesterol and LDL in the low-carbohydrate diets, with a significant elevation in HDL levels at both 6 months and 1 year of 4.6 mg/dl and 3.1 mg/dl, respectively. Triglycerides also showed a favorable response at 6 months and 1 year, with statistically significant decreases of 22 mg/dl and 31 mg/dl, respectively. The authors of this meta-analysis point out the attrition rate of 30% to 50% as a major limiting factor in the interpretation of these trials. Finally, the author reiterates the fact that there are no studies evaluating the effect of low-carbohydrate diets on cardiovascular morbidity and mortality [14]. This fact is a major impediment to making general recommendations for or against these particular diets for our patients.

Very Low Fat Diets

Very low fat diets have become an area of interest since the Seven Countries Study revealed a low risk of cardiovascular disease and increased longevity in a Japanese cohort who maintained a fat intake of 10% or less [15]. This interest was further bolstered by data in multiple animal and human studies that showed that a higher intake of saturated fat and cholesterol caused atherosclerosis. Furthermore, some investigators showed lower lipid levels in strict vegetarians during the 1970s [16]. Several authors have presented low-fat diets aimed toward the reduction of heart disease. Dean Ornish and Nathan Pritikin are the best known of these investigators [17,18]. Both these programs incorporate exercise, stress management, and a diet consisting of minimal dietary fat.

Both authors report regression of coronary disease utilizing their programs; however, the Ornish program has the best evidence to support these claims. His initial pilot study was a randomized, controlled trial of 46 ischemic heart disease patients who were randomized to stress management with an "essentially vegan diet" with the control group continuing their usual diet and activity [19]. The experimental group was housed in a "rural" environment with all meals provided to them. Stress management techniques were taught for 5 h per day. The diet did not contain salt, sugar, alcohol, or caffeine. Caloric intake was approximately 1400 kcal with 5.2 mg dietary cholesterol. Exercise was not a component of this study. The groups were followed for approximately 3 weeks. Baseline testing consisted of myocardial perfusion exercise testing, lipid panel testing, angina symptom frequency, and medication reporting. The experimental group showed increased exercise capacity and decreased total cholesterol (−20.5%), triglycerides (−20%), and HDL. The author did show that the HDL:total cholesterol ratio remained the same and notes that this may be more predictive of coronary risk in vegetarians. Anginal episodes decreased from 10 episodes per week to fewer than 1 episode in the experimental group. There was a trend toward improved cardiac wall motion and ejection fraction in the experimental group as well.

Building on these findings, Ornish and colleagues studied a larger number of ischemic heart patients, utilizing a more intensive program that included smoking cessation, a 10% fat, "whole foods vegetarian" diet, aerobic exercise, stress management training, and group psychosocial support [20]. These patients were studied for a period of 5 years and included 48 men and women. The main outcomes of this study were adherence to lifestyle changes and changes in coronary artery diameter stenosis and cardiac events. Secondary study endpoints were lipid levels, weight loss, and anginal frequency. Endpoints were evaluated at both 1 year and 5 years. The 28 patients in the intervention group showed the following after 5 years in the study:

1. A 20% decrease in LDL cholesterol versus 19% decrease in the control arm (60% of control patients were taking cholesterol-lowering medications while none of the experimental group took these medications).
2. No change in triglyceride or HDL levels between the groups.
3. A 7.9% increased coronary vessel diameter versus a 27% worsening in controls.
4. Increased BMI correlated with worsening progression of disease.
5. Anginal symptoms decreased by 72% after 5 years in experimental patients without intervention. The control group showed a 36% decrease, with 5 of 20 patients undergoing coronary angioplasty.

6. The experimental group was also shown to have improved perfusion during nuclear stress testing in a later study [21]. The control group had worsening coronary perfusion.

Criticism of these studies typically is aimed at the intensity of the program and difficulty with strict dietary adherence in a "free-living" environment. A Cochrane review was performed that evaluated 12 randomized, controlled trials which utilized low-fat diets in the treatment of obesity [22]. Trials ranged from 6 to 18 months. Weight loss and cholesterol levels *were not* noted to be significantly different at 1 year.

> **Conclusion:** For those willing to follow a stringent lifestyle plan, very low-fat diets and lifestyle changes offer some evidence of improvement in cardiovascular risk factors and outcomes. Adherence also shows lowering of LDL and HDL cholesterol levels.

Moderate Carbohydrate–High Protein Diets

The moderate carbohydrate–high protein diet is best exemplified by diets such as the The South Beach Diet, The Zone Diet, and other diets that focus on foods with a low glycemic index. The glycemic index is a measurement of serum blood glucose response to the ingestion of a 50-g portion of a given food item. Foods with a higher glycemic index cause a more rapid rise in the postprandial blood glucose levels over a 2-h period. The scale compares this carbohydrate load to the same load of a control food, usually glucose or white bread. In this way, the serum glucose responses to different foods are compared. In addition to a low glycemic index, most of these diets also emphasize the intake of "healthy fats" such as fish and olive oil [23,24]. These eating plans are based on the premise that a diet high in simple sugars or other high glycemic foods can cause high levels of circulating insulin. A long-term, hyperinsulinemic state is associated with the metabolic syndrome, a well-established risk factor profile for cardiovascular disease [2].

Diets marked by a high glycemic index have been correlated with unfavorable lipid profiles. The HDL of 14,907 participants of the NHANES (National Health and Nutrition Examination Survey) study was examined and correlated with the glycemic index of their diet based on food frequency questionnaires. A diet with a higher glycemic index was associated with lower HDL levels. This correlation persisted through multivariate analysis [25]. In contrast, a study of 335 randomly selected Danish men and women showed no significant relationship between lipid levels and glycemic index [26]. Although it is simple to measure the glycemic index of a single food, it becomes difficult to predict the response in items made of multiple foods. Furthermore, different populations show varied responses to glycemic load, which makes generalizations about a diet based on glycemic index difficult.

There are few randomized, controlled studies evaluating the aforementioned dietary approaches. Agatston, the author of the South Beach diet, compared his moderate-carbohydrate, high-protein diet to the National Cholesterol Education Program (NCEP) Step 2 diet in 60 men and women. The experimental diet consisted of 39% fat, 33% protein, and 28% low glycemic index carbohydrates, with 17% of the fat coming from a monounsaturated source, mainly olive oil. At the end of 12 weeks, dieters in the experimental arm showed greater weight loss, but no difference in lipid parameters, compared to the control group. There were no adverse outcomes in the experimental group [27].

A study comparing the Zone, Weight Watchers, the Ornish, and the Atkins diet was performed by Dansinger and colleagues [28]. In this study, 160 overweight or obese adults (BMI 27–42) with at least one cardiac risk factor were randomized to each of the four diets for a period of 1 year. Primary outcomes included dietary adherence, weight, BMI, waist circumference, total cholesterol, LDL cholesterol, HDL cholesterol, triglycerides, glucose, and blood pressure. Dietary adherence was low for all diets, with 35% to 50% of patients discontinuing their diet before 1 year. Although not reaching statistical significance, Atkins and Ornish had higher discontinuation rates than Weight Watchers and Zone. All the dieters lost moderate amounts of weight, with 10% of individuals losing more than 10% of their body weight. There was no difference in weight loss between the diets. All the diets except Atkins reduced LDL by a statistically significant amount at 1 year. All the diets raised HDL except for the Ornish diet. None of the diets significantly changed triglycerides, blood pressure, or fasting glucose. Of note, all the diets caused a statistically significant lowering of C-reactive protein, a known inflammatory marker in cardiovascular disease. Notably, none of the diets caused any adverse affects or significant worsening of cardiovascular risk factors. It should also be noted that the cardiovascular risk factor reductions seen are similar to those that would be expected with weight loss alone, except for the Atkins group, which did not show this reduction.

Conclusions: There are no patient- or disease- oriented data to recommend for or against the aforementioned diets; however, much of the dietary advice is borrowed from Mediterranean diet outcomes, which do decrease coronary risk. These diets deserve further long-term study.

The Mediterranean Diet

In 1970, the Seven Countries study was published, which described the mortality and dietary intakes in 16 cohorts from around the world. Great interest was sparked by the longevity of one cohort located on the isle of Crete, where fat intake was high, but cardiovascular mortality was paradoxically low [29]. The group included 12,763 men aged from 40 to 59 years old who were located in the United States, Finland, Croatia, the Netherlands, Italy, Greece, and Japan. Menotti et al. published data that followed these men over 25 years and looked at all-cause mortality. Risk factors and dietary intake were recorded in these cohorts. East Finland, the country with the highest intake of saturated fat, had the highest death rate from cardiovascular disease. The lowest death rates were seen in Crete and Belgrade, Serbia. Serum cholesterol was only predictive of mortality in some areas. This study spurred further evaluation of dietary patterns in the Mediterranean region of the world, especially in light of an increased relative fat intake of 35% to 40% of total calories [30].

Although the exact makeup of the Mediterranean diet is not standardized, it has several key components that include an increased intake of the following foods [31]:

1. Food derived from plant sources, including fruits, vegetables, breads, cereals, potatoes, legumes, and nuts
2. Fish and poultry
3. Up to four eggs per week
4. Locally grown, minimally processed food
5. Red wine in low to moderate amounts with meals
6. Daily dairy products in low to moderate amounts
7. Infrequent red meat intake
8. Olive oil as the principal source of fat
9. Desserts composed mainly of fresh fruits

As opposed to many of the previously mentioned studies, the Mediterranean diet has several disease-oriented, population-based studies to support its use. The Lyons Diet Heart Study was a prospective, randomized, single-blinded trial that evaluated the effectiveness of a Mediterranean diet on secondary prevention in patients with known cardiovascular disease. Three hundred patients were randomized after their first myocardial infarction to either a Mediterranean diet high in alpha-linoleic acid or a low-fat postinfarct diet. The initial results of the study, released after 27 months of follow-up, showed no difference in serum lipids, blood pressure, or BMI between the two groups. However, Mediterranean dieters showed a 73% relative risk reduction for fatal and nonfatal myocardial infarction. Overall mortality risk reduction was 70%. The same group of investigators followed these patients for a mean duration of 46 months. Dietary compliance was greater than 70%, with compliance measured utilizing food questionnaires and confirmed with serum alpha-linoleic acid measurements. Higher levels of serum alpha-linoleic acid were associated with improved outcomes. A Mediterranean diet provided a relative risk reduction of 47% to 72% in the following endpoints: myocardial infarction, angina, stroke, heart failure, pulmonary embolism, and deep venous thrombosis. These findings persisted independently of the following traditional risk factors: total cholesterol, systolic blood pressure, male sex, and aspirin use. There was no significant difference in the lipid profiles of the patients in the two groups. These findings suggested an independent cardioprotective mechanism of the Mediterranean diet in addition to typical risk factor reduction. The authors recommend a cardioprotective diet in addition to individual risk factor treatment [32]. These findings were replicated by the GISSI (Gruppo Italiano per lo Studio della Sopravvivenza nell'Infarto) investigators who showed that supplementation with n-3 polyunsaturated fatty acids after a myocardial infarction reduced the risk of recurrence, stroke, and death by 10%. The outcome difference between the groups was seen as soon as 3 months in this large study of more than 10,000 patients [33]. The same group of investigators showed a 49% risk reduction in repeat myocardial infarction after implementation of a traditional Mediterranean diet [34].

A similar trial by Singh and colleagues was undertaken to evaluate the effect of an Indo-Mediterranean diet in a South Asian population. The purpose of this randomized, single-blinded study was to evaluate the feasibility of adopting a Mediterranean-type diet to the South Asian population utilizing locally available sources of n-3 fatty acids to include soybean or mustard seed oil rather than the olive oil typically seen in a classic Mediterranean diet. One thousand patients over the age of 25 with coronary artery disease or coronary artery disease risk factors (hypercholesterolemia, hypertension, diabetes, angina, or previous myocardial infarction) were randomized to an NCEP Step 1 diet or a Mediterranean-style diet. All patients were counseled on exercise, smoking cessation, and stress relief. Endpoints included fatal and nonfatal myocardial infarction and sudden cardiac death. Approximately 54% of patients were taking aspirin, and 6% to 7% of patients took statin medications. After 2 years, the intervention group had lowered total cholesterol by approximately 21 mg/dl. More importantly, the intervention diet reduced the relative risk of nonfatal myocardial infarction by 53%, that of sudden cardiac death by 67%, and of fatal myocardial infarction by 33%. Fatal myocardial infarction reduction was the only endpoint that did not reach statistical significance [35]. These findings were described in free-living settings as well, where individuals purchased and prepared their own foods.

Trichopoulou and colleagues followed 22,043 Greek adults for 44 months. Adherence to a traditional Mediterranean diet led to a 25% all-cause mortality reduction, with a 33% reduction of coronary disease deaths [36].

Fat sources were compared by Estruch and colleagues, who published a large, blinded, randomized, controlled trial to evaluate three diets for 3 months: a low-fat diet, a Mediterranean diet supplemented with walnuts, and a Mediterranean diet supplemented with olive oil. The study group was considered high risk because of the presence of one or more coronary disease risk factors to include elevated LDL, decreased HDL, BMI greater than 25, or type 2 diabetes. This trial was a pilot study for the much larger PREDIMED trial (Prevencion con Dieta Mediterranea) that involved more than 9000 patients. The interventions included dietary counseling, with the low-fat dieters being given a copy of the American Health Association (AHA) guidelines and told to restrict fat to less than 30% of total intake. In contrast, the Mediterranean group was instructed in how to increase vegetable fats and oils. Participants were allocated an ample supply of olive oil and nuts each week. Most of the dieters were of European and Spanish descent. The following results were found:

1. Body weight was reduced in all three groups, with no significant differences between the groups.
2. C-reactive protein and other inflammatory markers were reduced in the Mediterranean diet group with olive oil, but remained unchanged in the low-fat and nut group.
3. Blood pressure was statistically lower in both Mediterranean groups.
4. Fasting glucose and insulin levels were lower in both Mediterranean groups.
5. Total cholesterol was lower in both Mediterranean groups in comparison to the low-fat group.
6. LDL was decreased by 3.4 to 3.9 mg/dl in comparison to the low-fat group.
7. HDL was increased by 1.6 to 2.9 mg/dl in comparison to the low-fat group.
8. Triglycerides were lowered by 7 to 13 mg/dl compared to the low-fat group.
9. More favorable changes were seen in the Mediterranean diet with nuts than in the diet with olive oil.

The authors point out that increased fat intake did not add to obesity measured by BMI, weight, and waist measurement. All cardiovascular risk factors were improved in the these participants [37].

Special Populations

Young Women

Lagio and colleagues studied 42,237 young women aged 30 to 49 years for a period of 12 years in Sweden. Adherence to a Mediterranean diet showed no difference in mortality rate in women under the age of 40, but there was a 13% reduction in overall mortality and 16% decrease in cancer mortality in patients over 40 who adhered to a Mediterranean style diet. There were very few deaths from coronary disease in this group of young women [38].

The Elderly

Knoops and colleagues evaluated the combined effects of the Mediterranean diet, physical activity, moderate alcohol use, and smoking on all-cause and specific cause mortality in apparently healthy men and women aged 70 to 90 years from 11 European countries. This study was part of the larger Healthy Aging in Europe Longitudinal Study (HALE). These individuals were followed for 12 years. A combination of Mediterranean diet, nonsmoking, moderate alcohol use, and increased physical activity correlated with a 65% decrease in overall mortality risk. Cardiovascular mortality was decreased by 61% [39].

Patients with Hypercholesterolemia With and Without Concomitant Use of Statins

Pitsavos and colleagues compared 848 coronary artery disease patients with 1078 cardiovascular disease-free controls; 63% of the patients with coronary artery disease had hypercholesterolemia compared with 37% of the controls. Treatment with a Mediterranean diet resulted in a 12% LDL reduction, while statin medications lowered LDL by 21%. Together, these factors reduced the risk of coronary disease by 43% in the control group. This finding suggests a risk reduction benefit *beyond that seen with a statin medication alone* [40].

The causes of the mortality benefits of the Mediterranean diet are debated. Diets rich in fruits and vegetables have been shown to reduce cardiovascular mortality in other populations [41]. Diets rich in omega-3 fatty acids have also been shown to decrease cardiovascular risk, with fish intake showing a dose-related decrease in risk beginning at one meal per week and increasing to five meals per week [42]. Although some investigators report a lack of effect on the markers of vascular inflammation, several studies support a decrease in plasma C-reactive protein, insulin level, and fasting blood glucose [43–46], known markers of inflammation that can predict coronary disease independent of plasma lipid levels.

This diet deserves study in modern Western populations to evaluate the difference between industrialized sources of agriculture to include eggs, fish, fruits, and vegetables. Some studies haves shown differing amounts of cardioprotective fats in eggs and cheese from animals in Greece, who may have different feed and grazing patterns.

The Mediterranean diet does offer patients a better-tasting, easier-to-follow alternative to traditional low-fat diets and likely confers cardiovascular benefits. Modifications to this diet could be applied to adapt it to different at-risk populations.

> **Conclusions:** The Mediterranean diet offers the best example of a long term dietary approach which appears to significantly reduce cardiovascular and overall mortality. Interestingly, these improvements occur with and without expected improvements in some traditional markers of cardiovascular risk such as LDL and blood pressure.

NCEP/TLC/AHA Dietary Guidelines

First introduced in 1993 in response to rising rates of coronary artery disease and data that supported healthy lipid profiles, the National Cholesterol Education Panel (NCEP) Step 1 and Step 2 diets have been frequently studied alone and in comparison to other dietary strategies. The goal of these diets was in line with the

U.S. Department of Health and Human Services goal to achieve total cholesterol of at least 200 in all Americans by the year 2000. Since that time, the guidelines have been modified and replaced with the Therapeutic Lifestyle Change, or TLC, in 2000 to incorporate recently elucidated information about coronary risk [47]. These guidelines were incorporated into a broader set of recommendations in 2006 released by the American Heart Association (AHA) and deemed the Diet and Lifestyle Recommendations Revision 2006 [48].

It is useful to look at the historical basis and patient-oriented results of the NCEP guidelines implementation to better understand and utilize the current TLC and AHA recommendations. There are no new prospective studies utilizing the latter set of guidelines because of their relatively recent publication. Furthermore, the breadth of the recommendations makes these interventions difficult to study in a free-living population while utilizing a randomized, controlled framework.

NCEP Step 1 and Step 2 Overview

The NCEP Step 1 diet was designed to lower the dietary intake of saturated fat and cholesterol, with a goal of decreasing LDL by 7% to 9%. This goal was achieved by limiting total dietary fat to less than 30%, saturated fat to less than 10%, and dietary cholesterol to less than 300 mg per day. If cholesterol goals were not met with this approach, the more stringent Step 2 diet decreased saturated fat to less than 7% and dietary cholesterol to less than 300 mg per day. The Step 2 diet was expected to lower LDL cholesterol by 10% to 20%. The guidelines also recommend a diet rich in fruits, vegetables, whole grains, low-fat dairy products, lean meats, and fish.

In a summary statement by the American Heart Association, it was noted that "Many Americans will be unable to achieve the maximal cholesterol lowering potential expected of these dietary recommendations and thus will require pharmacologic intervention [49]." This group commented further on the probable benefit of plant sterols, dietary fiber, and a high HDL cholesterol level. They recommended that many individuals should follow these diets, with an emphasis on patients with diabetes and those with known coronary disease.

The NCEP diets have been studied extensively in several settings. The following studies highlight the benefits and limitations of this diet.

NCEP Diet Alone and Cardiovascular Risk Factors

Yu-Poth and colleagues performed a meta-analysis on 37 trials utilizing the NCEP Step 1 and 2 diets, with a focus on combined outcomes on cardiovascular disease risk factors. This study only evaluated trials that utilized "free-living" participants, meaning that they had to purchase and prepare their own meals. The investigators thought that this criterion provided a better reflection of treatment interventions in the general population. They found that that the Step 1 diet favorably reduced total cholesterol, LDL, and triglycerides by 10%, 12%, and 8%, respectively. Step 2 reduced these same values by 13%, 16%, and 8%. A Step 1 diet did not decrease HDL; however, the lower fat/saturated fat Step 2 diet was found to decrease HDL by 7%. Regression analysis showed that for every 1% decrease in saturated fat intake, total cholesterol decreased by 2.2 mg/dl and LDL decreased by 1.95 mg/dl. The researchers also confirmed a correlation between body weight and lipid profiles. A 1-kg decrease in body weight correlated with a decrease in triglycerides of 0.97 mg/dl and an increase in HDL of 0.42 mg/dl. They also found that exercise resulted in greater decreases in total cholesterol, LDL, and triglycerides while preventing the HDL decrease usually seen in low-fat diets [50]. Unfavorable HDL changes with an isocaloric NCEP diet were also noted by Walden et al., who showed 8% LDL lowering over a 6-month period, but decreases in HDL of 4% to 6% in women and 1% to 3% in men [51]. These findings were replicated in other settings utilizing a hypocaloric version of the diet as well [52,53].

Conclusion: The NCEP Step 1 and 2 diets are effective at improving serum LDL levels, but may have deleterious effects on HDL cholesterol levels.

NCEP with or Without Exercise

In 1991, before the release of the actual guidelines, Wood et al. compared the effects of a hypocaloric NCEP Step 1 diet with and without exercise with a control group that continued its regular dietary intake for 1 year. This group of 264 men and women, who were 25 to 49 years old, lost significant weight utilizing the NCEP diet and reached LDL reduction goals of 7% to 9%. However, the group that did not exercise actually saw decreases in HDL cholesterol; this effect was greater in women than men. HDL levels increased in the group that maintained a hypocaloric, Step 1 diet in combination with exercise. This finding supported the necessity of exercise in combination with a diet low in fat and cholesterol. No disease-oriented endpoints were reported [54].

The same group of investigators studied 377 men and women with low HDL (less than 59 mg/dl in women, less than 44 mg/dl in men) and moderately elevated LDL (more than 125 mg/dl but less than 210 mg/dl in women; more than 125 mg/dl but less than 190 mg/dl in men). The subjects were randomly assigned to four groups: NCEP Step 2 diet alone, exercise alone (3 h/week of aerobic activity), NCEP Step 2 plus exercise, and a control group that utilized the NCEP Step 1 diet. Endpoints included body weight and lipid profiles after 1 year. NCEP Step 2 dieters lost weight, decreased dietary intake of cholesterol and saturated fat, but did not change their HDL or LDL levels in comparison to the control group (NCEP Step 1). The group that undertook *diet and exercise* had the most beneficial changes, with decreased LDL and weight. HDL levels did not differ significantly among the groups [55].

NCEP Step 1 and 2 and Cardiovascular Outcomes

There are relatively few studies that focus on the NCEP diet and cardiovascular endpoints. Investigators from the Women's Health Initiative performed a randomized, controlled prospective trial on 48,835 postmenopausal women. The intervention group underwent dietary intervention to include group and individual behavioral modification sessions that focused on a low-fat (less than 20%) diet, increased intake of fruits and vegetables (at least five servings/day), and increased intake of grains (at least six servings/day). The control group received diet-related education materials. The behavior modification group lowered their dietary fat intake by 8.2% after 6 years of follow-up. Of note, decreases were seen in all fat type intakes to include saturated, monounsaturated, and polyunsaturated fats. Fruit and vegetable intake was increased by an average of one serving per day compared to controls. Grains were increased by 0.5 intakes per day. It was not noted whether this intake included whole and processed grains. LDL levels were reduced in the intervention group by 3.5 mg/dl. Stroke, fatal, and nonfatal myocardial infarction incidence did not differ significantly between the groups during the 8 years of follow-up. There was a trend toward decreased coronary disease in groups stratified to lower saturated fat and greater fruit and vegetable intake.

The study group commented that the intake of polyunsaturated fat, fruit, vegetables, and fiber was lower than is currently recommended [56]. It should be mentioned that the fat intake of this diet was also significantly lower than is recommended by the NCEP diet, which could have led to decreased HDL levels and a negative impact on cardiovascular risk.

Conclusion: There is a paucity of disease oriented outcome data to recommend for or against a low fat diet, NCEP Step 1 and 2 diets.

NCEP Diet Compliance

The NCEP diet has been used as a control/comparison in multiple study settings, with compliance rates comparable to other dietary plans. Large studies looking specifically at compliance are lacking, although the aforementioned Women's Health Initiative group studied compliance to the NCEP diet in 13,777 hypercholesterolemic women who also required drug therapy. Only 20% of these women reported compliance with the dietary recommendations. Interestingly, the subsample reporting compliance had *higher* LDL levels. Patients who reported higher levels of compliance were more likely to have suffered a prior cardiovascular event. Compliance was also associated with fruit and vegetable intake and a higher education level.

Obesity, smoking, marriage, and a sedentary lifestyle were all associated with lower compliance rates [57].

Conclusion: Compliance to NCEP diet recommendations is poor in a high risk population. Compliance was not necessarily associated with improved LDL levels.

NCEP Diet with Supplementation

Several small studies have been performed that examined the effects of supplementing or replacing ingredients of a typical NCEP diet. Jenkins et al. examined 20 patients receiving an NCEP Step 2 diet that was then augmented with soy protein and soluble fiber. The resultant diet increased HDL cholesterol levels by 6.4%, in contrast to the decreased HDL levels that have been mentioned previously. Oxidized LDL levels were also lower in the test group [58]. Another group investigated patients receiving the NCEP Step 2 diet with and without supplementation with fish fatty acids. This small study of 22 patients showed greater decreases in LDL and total cholesterol among the fish fatty acid group, but also found that HDL was lowered by an additional 6 percentage points (–11% versus –17%). Of note, postprandial triglyceride levels were lower in the fish group [59]. NCEP dieters who ingested cereals that were high in fiber, in particular, psyllium, were shown to have additional LDL cholesterol-lowering benefits. Triglycerides and HDL were not affected [60].

Conclusion: Supplementation of the NCEP Step 2 diet with fiber, soy protein, or fish fatty acids may lead to improved lipid profiles. No disease oriented endpoints were reported in these studies.

From NCEP to TLC

The advent of the NCEP dietary guidelines ushered in an era of fat consciousness and low fat food intake, but it brought about a set of incomplete guidelines with regard to overall coronary risk. The restriction of dietary fat led to a shift in food content and dietary intake to foods with "low fat" but higher sugar content. Further research also emerged that refuted pure fat restriction, but instead advocated a diet of fat substitution. In 2001, the National Heart, Lung, and Blood Institute released the Therapeutic Lifestyle Changes plan (TLC) designed for people at higher risk for heart disease; these guidelines were designed to replace the NCEP Step 2 guidelines. Several studies were released after the original NCEP report to support the additions and changes implemented in the TLC guidelines.

Fatty Acids: Dietary Fat Impact on Coronary Risk and Lipids

Before discussing dietary fats and their impact on cardiovascular disease, it is useful to review the different types of fats and their common source in the diet. Table 3.2 describes the most commonly studied dietary fats and their most common sources. This table lists the "good" and "bad" fats with regard to coronary artery disease to assist healthcare providers in giving specific recommendations to their patients.

Hu and colleagues studied the dietary intake of 80,082 healthy young women aged 34 to 59 years for 14 years by a validated food intake questionnaire. Of these patients, 939 experienced a fatal myocardial infarction (MI) or death from coronary artery disease. The investigators studied nutrient intake and found that an increase in saturated fat intake by 5% versus the same amount in carbohydrates resulted in a 17% increase in the risk of coronary artery disease. *trans* saturated fatty acids caused a 93% risk increase for every increase of 2% in intake. In contrast, an increase of 5% in the dietary intake of monounsaturated fats decreased risk by 19%. Polyunsaturated fat showed an even more impressive 38% relative risk reduction in this large cohort [61]. This study suggested that fat type rather than fat amount was at least partially responsible for heart disease prevention. These results were validated by repeated studies and large meta-analyses that showed that *trans* saturated fatty acids adversely effected lipid profiles [62,63].

Fruit and Vegetable Intake

Although population-based studies suggested that an increased intake of fruits and vegetables improved cardiovascular risk, few large studies unequivocally supported this until the late 1990s and early 2000s. In 2001, Joshipura et al. published a prospective cohort study that combined the data from the Nurses Health Study (84,251 women aged 34–59 years old) and the Health Professionals Follow-up Study (42,148 men aged 40–70 years old). The dietary intake of the women and men was followed for 14 years and 8 years, respectively. All the participants were free of known coronary disease, cancer, and diabetes mellitus at baseline.

Table 3.2 Fatty acids and their sources

Fat type	Derived from
Monounsaturated fatty acids (MUFA)	Olive oil and canola oil
Polyunsaturated fatty acids (PUFA)	Safflower, corn, soybean, flaxseed, sesame, and sunflower oils; fatty fish (omega-3), nuts
Saturated fatty acids (unfavorable)	Mainly animal/dairy fat; hydrogenated MUFA/PUFA
trans fatty acids (unfavorable)	Industrially hydrogenated vegetable oils; fried foods; animal fats

After adjustment for known cardiovascular risk factors to include smoking, hypertension, and family history, fruit and vegetable intake accounted for a 20% decrease in the highest quintile intake group as compared with the lowest intake cohort. Each single serving of fruits and vegetables (more than four servings) accounted for a 4% lower relative risk of coronary heart disease. The greatest protective effect was seen by those ingesting the largest amounts of green leafy vegetables, vitamin C-rich fruits, and vegetables. Potatoes, legumes, and fruit juice did not show the same protective benefits. Decreased risk began at four servings per day with the most significant protection occurring at eight or more servings per day. The protective effect was greater in current smokers than in former or nonsmokers. The authors attributed the beneficial effects as resulting from fiber, antioxidants, vitamins, and potassium. The authors compare the 20% event risk reduction rate to the 30% risk reduction seen with statin medications and note that the combined effects could be additive [64].

Another large study examining healthy eating patterns was published by Hu et al. in 2000. This study, of 44,875 healthy men aged 40 to 75 years, compared cardiovascular outcomes in a group eating a mainly "Western" diet consisting of a higher intake of red meat, processed meat, refined grains, simple carbohydrates, fried foods, and high-fat dairy products with a group consuming a prudent diet that consisted of a higher intake of fruits and vegetables, whole grains, legumes, fish, and poultry. After adjustment for age and traditional coronary artery disease (CAD) risk factors, it was shown that those who followed a "prudent diet" had a 30% relative risk reduction of CAD, whereas those who followed a typical "Western" diet had a 64% increased relative risk of CAD [65]. A similar study was repeated in women by the same group of investigators. Risk reductions were similar, with a 24% reduction and 46% increase, respectively [66].

Steffen et al. studied whole-grain, fruit, and vegetable intake and found that whole grains conferred similar benefits in all patients. In contrast to other studies, fruit and vegetable intake did not confer a significant benefit in white patients. However, there was a benefit in black patients with an increased intake of fruits and vegetables [67]. Data from the National Health and Nutrition Examination Survey released in 2002 showed similar results with regard to heart disease and stroke. This data set encompassed 9,608 adults aged 25 to 74 years over a 19-year period. Consumption of fruits and vegetables three times per day as compared with one time per day resulted in a 27% decrease in stroke, a 42% lower stroke mortality, and a 24% lower ischemic heart disease mortality, *after* adjustment for cardiovascular risk factors [41].

Conclusion: Increased intake of fruit, vegetables, and whole grains reduces cardiovascular morbidity and mortality.

Therapeutic Lifestyle Changes

The complete Therapeutic Lifestyle Changes diet can be found on the National Heart, Lung, and Blood Institute web page (www.nhlbi.nih.gov) as a part of the Adult Treatment Panel III Recommendations for the Treatment of Hyperlipidemia. These recommendations are part of a multipronged approach that focus on individual and population change. The dietary changes are prescribed for a total of 6 weeks before reevaluation of lipid levels and assessment for medication needs. It is recommended that dietary intervention continue as long as progress is being made toward the patient's goal LDL. LDL goals are based on individual patient risks. The website serves as a good reference point for patients and healthcare workers looking for specific examples of soluble fiber and heart-healthy foods. The guidelines focus on interventions that are known to lower LDL levels and increase HDL levels. A synopsis of the guidelines follows [47]:

1. LDL increases approximately 2% for every 1% increase in dietary saturated fat. Reduction of saturated fat intake has been shown to decrease LDL levels by as much as 8%. LDL cholesterol remains the main focus of these guidelines. This is one factor that differentiates them from the new AHA lifestyle guidelines.
2. Weight reduction alone will reduce LDL regardless of nutrient composition of the weight loss plan, but a diet that is lower in saturated fat and cholesterol will enhance and sustain LDL lowering. Multiple studies of hypocaloric diets confirm this finding [28].
3. High intakes of saturated fatty acids are associated with high rates of coronary disease within populations.
4. *trans* fatty acids can raise serum LDL cholesterol levels. Intake should be kept to a minimum.
5. Dietary cholesterol should be kept to 200 mg/day or less.
6. Monounsaturated fatty acids (MUFA) lower LDL cholesterol if they replace saturated fatty acids; these do not lower HDL or raise triglycerides. Controlled clinical trials have not examined the coronary disease outcomes of these fatty acids; they can comprise up to 20% of total calories.
7. Polyunsaturated fatty acids (PUFA) consisting of mainly n-6 linoleic acid reduce LDL when substituted for saturated fatty acids. They can also lower HDL at high doses. Some large trials show that some cardiovascular disease endpoints can be lowered by this substitution. PUFA can equal 10% of total calories [31,68].
8. It is *not* necessary to restrict total fat if fat intake guidelines minimizing saturated and *trans* fat intake are followed.
9. Carbohydrates should be kept under 60% of total intake because of increased risk of lowering HDL cholesterol and increasing serum triglycerides.
10. Dietary protein has little effect on serum cholesterol.
11. Soluble fiber, 5–10 g per day, reduces LDL cholesterol levels by 5%.

12. Plant stanols at 2–3 g per day can lower LDL by 6%–15%.
13. High intakes of soy protein may lower LDL.
14. Omega-3 (n-3) fatty acids such as soybean oil, canola oil, walnuts, flaxseed oil, and fish oil can decrease coronary heart disease risk. These data are compiled mainly from the Mediterranean diet studies [29–40,42–46,68,69].
15. The recommended daily allowance of 400 μg folate should be taken. Data are not sufficient to support the treatment of hyperhomocystenemia with folate supplementation.
16. A diet low in salt is recommended.
17. Antioxidants are not recommended.
18. High-fat, high-protein diets are not recommended.

Conclusions: The above recommendations can result in LDL lowering of 20–30 percent, although some would surmise a greater amount of risk reduction from these guidelines based on non-LDL risk factor modification (47).

The DASH Diet

The new American Heart Association Diet and Lifestyle revisions reference the TLC or DASH diets as integral components to their lifestyle plan. The DASH, or Dietary Approaches to Stop Hypertension Eating Plan, has been validated in randomized controlled studies with high-risk patient populations such as those with the metabolic syndrome. This diet has many similarities to the NCEP Step 2 diet, except for a 2.4 g/day sodium restriction, and has been shown to increase HDL and lower triglycerides, systolic blood pressure, fasting blood glucose, and weight [70].

The American Heart Association Diet and Lifestyle Recommendations Revision Revision 2006 [71]

Released in the summer of 2006, these guidelines are aimed at overall lifestyle versus diet alone in the prevention of coronary artery disease. They were released to reflect new evidence that shows risk reduction in addition to that shown by LDL or HDL treatment alone. Furthermore, the guidelines were written to be more easily understood by patient and healthcare providers with an emphasis on practical approaches to implementation. These recommendations include overcoming commonly encountered difficulties including incorporation of sound food choices when eating out. Finally, the guidelines focus on a larger population by targeting schools, healthcare professionals, the food industry, and restaurants for their role in educating the general public about obesity prevention and healthy eating.

The obesity epidemic is recognized as a major risk factor for cardiovascular disease. A synopsis of the guidelines follows. Similarities to the therapeutic lifestyle changes exist, but attempts have been made at simplification.

General Goals

1. Consume an overall healthy diet: The guidelines cite numerous dietary patterns, such as the Mediterranean diet, which show a decrease in cardiovascular disease and risk factors. A "whole diet" emphasis is made rather than an emphasis on specific nutrients. The following specific recommendations are made:

   a. Balance calories with physical intake to maintain a healthy body weight.
   b. Consume a diet rich in fruits, vegetables, whole grain, and fiber.
   c. Consume oily fish at least two times per week.
   d. Limit intake of saturated fatty acids to less than 7% of total intake per day and *trans* fatty acids to less than 1% per day. Total cholesterol intake should be limited to less than 300 mg per day.
   e. Achieve the previous goal by choosing lean meats and vegetable alternatives, using fat-free and low-fat dairy products, and minimizing intake of hydrogenated fat.
   f. Minimize the intake of foods or beverages with high or added sugar.
   g. Choose and prepare foods with little salt.
   h. If you drink alcohol, do so in moderation.
   i. When you eat outside the home, follow these same recommendations.

2. Aim for a healthy body weight:

   a. Achieve a BMI of 18.5 to 24.9 kg/m [2].
   b. Two-thirds of adults are overweight or obese.
   c. Obesity is an independent risk factor for cardiovascular disease.
   d. The obesity epidemic is multifactorial with a combination of increased caloric food density, sedentary lifestyle, and increased access to cheap, plentiful food.
   e. Increased emphasis should be put on weight gain prevention as weight loss is more difficult than prevention of gain.

3. Aim for recommended levels of LDL, HDL, and triglycerides:

   a. Increasing LDL levels increases the risk of cardiovascular disease. *trans* fatty acids increase LDL as much as saturated fatty acids; however, saturated fatty acids increase HDL levels whereas *trans* fats do not; this is thought to explain some of the increased risk of *trans* fats.
   b. The HDL level is inversely related to the risk of cardiovascular disease. Low HDL is associated with diabetes, hypertriglyceridemia, very low fat diets, and obesity.
   c. Triglycerides should be maintained at less than 150 mg/dl, and HDL should be above 40 mg/dl in men and above 50 mg/dl in women.

4. Aim for a normal blood pressure:

   a. Risk of cardiovascular disease increases as the blood pressure exceeds 120/80 mmHg. A decrease in salt intake and calories coupled with increases in fruit and vegetable intake as well as moderate alcohol consumption has been shown to lower blood pressure values.

5. Aim for a normal glucose level:

   a. Fasting blood glucose should be maintained below 100 mg/dl.

6. Maintain regular physical activity:

   a. Sixty-one percent of adults do not engage in regular physical activity. Sixty minutes of exercise most days of the week is recommended for weight loss. Thirty minutes of exercise on most days of the week is recommended to maintain weight and cardiovascular benefits.

7. Avoid use of or exposure to tobacco products.

Dietary specifics of the new AHA guidelines are more specific than previously released recommendations and incorporate findings of many of the previously mentioned studies in this chapter as well as specific lifestyle guidelines. The authors are quick to point out that these guidelines encompass an overall healthy lifestyle change aimed at reducing cardiovascular disease, not a diet to be followed with a specific goal such as weight loss or LDL lowering. These guidelines were also developed for healthy eating in all age groups except for those under the age of 2 years. The group recognizes that risk factors for obesity and cardiovascular disease are appearing at an earlier age, which is attributed to decreased physical activity, increased portion sizes, and increased caloric content of food served and marketed to and for children.

Specific Dietary Recommendations

1. Individuals should increase their knowledge of food calorie content. This understanding will aid in prevention of weight gain and assist with a hypocaloric diet plan in those attempting to lose weight.
2. Consume a diet rich in fruits and vegetables. As noted from the studies already described, this dietary change can lower the risk of cardiovascular disease [41,64–67]. Deeply colored fruits and vegetables are recommended as they are higher in micronutrient content. Fruit juice is not a suitable replacement for fruit. An increase in dietary fruits and vegetables lowers the energy density of the diet while increasing both soluble and nonsoluble fiber.
3. Choose whole-grain, high-fiber foods. This change increases the diet quality and decreases the risk of coronary artery disease by a modest reduction of LDL, accomplished through viscous or soluble fiber intake. This LDL lowering is in addition to that achieved by a diet low in saturated or *trans* fatty acids. Insoluble fiber intake has been shown to decrease cardiovascular disease as well. It may also slow gastric emptying, leading to increased satiety and decreased caloric intake. One-half of grain intake should come from whole grains.

4. Consume oily fish at least two times per week. The omega-3 fatty acids found in oily fish decrease the risk of sudden death from coronary artery disease. They may also displace foods that are higher in *trans* and saturated fatty acid. Frying fish can cause unhealthy *trans* isomerization of oils, which may negate the positive effects associated with fish intake. Intake of fish by pregnant women or children should be undertaken with caution because of concerns about water contaminants.

5. Limit the intake of saturated and *trans* fatty acids. Saturated fat should be limited to 7% or less of the daily dietary intake; this is in line with previous dietary guidelines. *trans* fatty acids should be limited to less than 1% of dietary intake. This goal should be easier to follow in the United States as of January 2006, when food labels began containing mandatory labeling regarding saturated and *trans* fat contents. The current mean U.S. intake of saturated fat is 11.2%; mean *trans* fat intake is 2.7%. Most saturated fat is derived from animal sources. *trans* fat is found in fried food and baked goods. Recommended strategies to accomplish this goal include low-fat substitution of dairy products and increased intake of fish, lean meats, and beans. Total fat intake has been liberalized and can be kept at 25% to 35% as long as those ingesting the upper limit do so with monounsaturated and polyunsaturated fats.

6. Minimize intake of sugar and high-sugar foods. Many foods marketed as low fat contain large amounts of simple sugars to improve flavor. These foods increase the caloric density of the foods and contribute to lower HDL cholesterol levels and to obesity as well [25].

7. Decrease overall salt intake to assist with blood pressure control.

8. Limit alcohol use to two drinks per day for men and one drink per day for women.

9. Be aware of the nutrient makeup of food prepared outside the home.

10. Antioxidant supplements are not recommended.

11. Soy protein studies have been inconclusive, but soy protein-rich foods may decrease cardiovascular risk when they replace animal and dairy products.

12. There is no evidence for folate or vitamin B supplementation.

13. No conclusive evidence is available regarding phytochemicals.

14. Fish oil supplementation is recommended for patients with coronary artery disease at a dose of 1 g/day. This intake can also be accomplished through the intake of oily fish in the diet.

15. Plant stanols and sterols may be used for additional LDL-lowering benefits of up to 15%.

16. Lifestyle guidance should be started in children as young as 2 years old.

17. Metabolic syndrome patients should avoid a very low fat diet as it may exacerbate low HDL and elevated triglyceride levels.

18. Dietary interventions are helpful in slowing the progression of chronic kidney disease.

19. The AHA recommends ethnically sensitive dietary changes, taking into consideration a patient's cultural dietary background and available foods when implementing dietary changes [71].

These guidelines incorporate evidence from many of the dietary trials accomplished in the last decade. They include most of the dietary interventions with a sound evidence basis and are an attempt at a more inclusive dietary plan as opposed to a restrictive program that focuses on limitations. Further study of these recommendations and their impact on food labeling, advertising, and intake is warranted. Clinical outcome studies that focus on cardiovascular disease and compliance will be of further utility for practicing clinicians.

Summary Recommendations

The aforementioned dietary guidelines and studies offer clinicians a large array of choices to utilize in frontline patient care. This array of choices can be overwhelming to both patients and healthcare providers. Furthermore, healthcare providers often find themselves in a time- and resource-limited environment. Optimally, all patients with *any* cardiovascular risk factors would be offered standardized dietary counseling and follow-up. However, formal dietary counseling and follow-up is time- and resource intensive and is therefore typically limited to those patients with the highest risk, such those with known coronary disease and diabetics. This approach, although somewhat effective, misses the goal of early primary prevention in the larger population at hand. Therefore, effective strategies for population and individual dietary counseling and therapy must be improved to reach the increasing number of at-risk patients. This goal will need to be accomplished in a stepwise progression with both healthcare providers and patients.

First and foremost, healthcare professionals need to educate themselves regarding diet and cardiovascular health. Effective counseling depends on a clinician's ability to translate sometimes cryptic dietary guidelines into real-world strategies for patients. Furthermore, providers need to learn how to adapt different dietary strategies to different racial and ethnic populations. Although many of the aforementioned diets have merit, the American Heart Association's guidelines offer the best conglomeration of goals and intervention that are both simple and generalizable.

Healthcare professionals need to seize upon all opportunities for lifestyle advice when faced with patients who exhibit any risk factors, to include obesity, hypertension, diabetes, or a strong family history of coronary disease. An assessment of patient readiness to change, learning style, and resources is an important part of this intervention. Once these factors are considered, a clinician should enact recommendations in a simple, stepwise fashion with attainable realistic goals. *Newer dietary strategies should emphasize what foods to include rather than listing all the foods to exclude.* It may be more clinically effective to offer patients a list of foods that they must eat each day, rather than giving them a longer list of foods that are forbidden. Most of the diets discussed in this chapter can provide some cardiovascular benefits. Patient lipid profile, preference, ethnicity, and socioeconomic background all play a part in their choice of diet. Tables 3.3 and 3.4 offer a brief summarization of the diets covered in this chapter. The greatest risk reduction will be accomplished if the diet chosen most closely follows your patient's individual preferences. The following

Table 3.3 Dietary components of diets discussed

Diet	Commercial examples	Calorie restriction?	Fat intake	Fruit/vegetable intake	Saturated/*trans* fat intake	Challenges
Low carbohydrate [4–9]	Atkins	No	Unlimited	Severe restriction	Unlimited, but discouraged	Urine ketone monitoring
Very low fat [13,17,19–21]	Ornish, Pritikin	No	Less than 10%	Vegetarian-based diet	None	Meditation, vegan diet, smoking cessation
TLC [47]	n/a	No	Less than 30%	High intake of "viscous fiber"	Less than 7%/ limit *trans* fat	Broad guidelines
AHA [71]	n/a	No	Unlimited	A diet "rich" in fruits and vegetables"	Less than 7%/ less than 1%	Broad guidelines
Low glycemic index/moderate carbohydrate [23,24,25,26,28]	South Beach, Zone, Sugar Busters	No	Unlimited	Limited	Limited	Glycemic index knowledge
Mediterranean [29–40, 42–46,68,69]	n/a	No	Unlimited	Encouraged	Limited	Costly, limited in some populations

TLC, therapeutic lifestyle charge; AHA, American Heart Association.

Table 3.4 Brief conclusions of diets discussed

Diet	Conclusion
Low carbohydrate [7–9]	No clinical outcomes or long-term data; may help high triglycerides and low HDL
Very low fat [13,17,19–21]	Impressive perfusion improvements, symptom reductions in a severely strict diet; lowers HDL
TLC [47]	A large group of guidelines that have proven LDL and cardiovascular benefits; application to "real world" patients deserves study
AHA [71]	Same as TLC, but with a greater emphasis on overall cardiovascular risk reduction and population health improvements
Moderate carbohydrates/low GI [23,24,25,26,28]	Offers sound principles without ample data
Mediterranean [29–40,42–46,68,69]	Excellent mortality data, but limited study populations

GI, glycemic index.

Table 3.5 Lifestyle interventions: clinical recommendations

Lifestyle intervention	Lipid profile improvement data	Morbidity/mortality benefit data
Count calories: achieve a hypocaloric diet for weight loss	Yes	Yes
Increase aerobic exercise to 30 min or more on most days; increase to 60 min for weight loss	Yes	Yes
Increase intake of "good" fats such as olive oil, canola oil, and nuts	Yes	Yes
Increase fresh fruits and vegetables	Yes	Yes
Increase whole-grain/high-fiber foods	Yes	Unknown
Consume oily fish twice per week	Yes	Yes
Limit saturated and *trans* fatty acids	Yes	Yes
Minimize sugar intake	Yes	Unknown
Limit salt intake to 2 g/day	No	Yes (with high BP)
Limit alcohol intake to two drinks per day for men and one for women	No	Yes[a]
Exercise caution when eating outside the home	Unknown	Unknown
Consider plant stanol supplementation	Yes	Unknown
Add omega-3 supplementation for those unable to eat fish	Yes	Unknown

BP, blood pressure.

[a] Alcohol abstinence may increase cardiovascular risk.

Source: Data from Lichtenstein A, Appel L, Brands M, Carnethon M, Daniels S, Franch H, Franklin B, Kris-Etherton P, Harris W, Howard B, Karanja N, Lefevre M, Rudel L, Sacks F, Van Horn L, Winston M, Wylie-Rosett J. AHA UPDATE: diet and lifestyle recommendations revision 2006. A scientific statement from the American Heart Association Nutrition Committee. Circulation 2006;114:82–96.

five-step plan offers a simple approach that can be utilized in an outpatient clinic setting without a large amount of ancillary support:

1. Make *one* significant dietary recommendation to your patients per visit. Multiple recommendations tend to be nonspecific and overwhelming. Spend time

explaining the proposed change and give the patients a written recommendation to post on their refrigerator or kitchen wall. Elicit feedback about the success of each intervention at subsequent visits. When one habit is formed, you can move on to the next recommendation.

2. Give your patients a web link or a written copy of specific dietary guidelines such as the AHA guidelines, the DASH diet, or the TLC recommendations. Utilize these guidelines as a basis for your recommendations. Highlight the specific

PATIENT NAME:_____

PATIENT DATE OF BIRTH:_____

My Lifestyle Changes	Lab Test	Result (Goal)	Date of Test	Change from Last Measurement
Eat fruits and vegetables before each meal	LDL	189 (130)	1/2/2007	
Stop smoking	HDL	35 (50)	1/2/2007	
Eat fish two times per week.	Triglycerides	240 (200)	1/2/2007	
Start cholesterol medication	HgA1C	8.0 (6.5)	1/2/2007	
	Blood Pressure	142/96 (130/80)	1/2/2007	
	Weight	231 (185)	1/2/2007	
	Daily Exercise Time	0 (30 minutes)	1/2/2007	
	Waist circumference	40 inches (34 inches)	1/2/2007	
	C-reactive protein	Not done	1/2/2007	
	Number of medications	5 (Zero!)	1/2/2007	

Fig. 3.1 Sample of patient report card

recommendations that you give them. The AHA guidelines incorporate many of the beneficial aspects of diets such as the Mediterranean diet and the NCEP Step 2 diet. These steps can be utilized as a roadmap toward cardiovascular health (Table 3.5).

3. Create a nutrition and lifestyle "report card" for your patients that contains their blood pressure, LDL, BMI, hemoglobin A1C, and Framingham risk along with specific goals for each of these parameters (Fig. 3.1). This report can be updated at each visit by you or your office staff to help encourage change. It is also useful to list specific interventions on this report card aimed at each of these parameters. Patients should be participants in filling out this report card with current values and a list of current goals.

4. Encourage patients to start every meal with fresh fruits or vegetables. This strategy will work toward the goal of ingesting more than five servings of these foods per day. These high-fiber, low caloric density foods will also help displace unhealthy foods eaten later in the meal. This single intervention is also a universal aspect of every successful cardiovascular risk reduction diet. Patients can accomplish this by ordering salads and fresh fruits while eating out. They may need to change shopping patterns, with more frequent market visits to obtain fresh fruits and vegetables.

5. Analyze each patient's dietary intake by asking him/her to document all food intake for a period of 1 week or more. This intervention exposes dietary pitfalls such as meal skipping or overindulgence in high-calorie beverages. It also provides a specific framework for feedback, rather than a "one size fits all" approach. A patient's reluctance to complete this task might also signal important issues with lifestyle change resistance or noncompliance.

A synopsis of the AHA dietary guidelines is available in Table 3.5. This table offers the busy clinician a quick list of possible interventions to utilize in the examination room.

References

1. NCHS E-stats: http://www.cdc.gov/nchs/products/pubs/pubd/hestats/obese/obse99.htm
2. Grundy SM, Brewer HB Jr, Cleeman JI, Smith SC Jr, Lenfant C, for the American Heart Association and National Heart, Lung, and Blood Institute. Definition of metabolic syndrome: report of the National Heart, Lung, and Blood Institute/American Heart Association conference on scientific issues related to definition. Circulation 2004;109:433–438.
3. Amazon.com search for "diet" books.
4. Atkins RC. Dr. Atkins' new diet revolution. New York: Simon & Schuster, 1998.
5. Yancy WS, Olsen MK, Guyton JR, Bakst RP, Westman EC. A low-carbohydrate, ketogenic diet versus a low-fat diet to treat obesity and hyperlipidemia. Ann Intern Med 2004;140: 769–777.
6. Foster GD, Wyatt HR, Hill, JO, McGuckin BG, Brill C, Mohammed BS, Szapary PO, Rader DJ, Edman JS, Klein S. A randomized trial of a low-carbohydrate diet for obesity. N Engl J Med 2003;348:2082–2090.
7. Samaha FF, Nayyar I, Prakash S, Chicano KL, Daily DA, McGrory, J, Williams T, Williams M, Gracely EJ, Stern L. A low-carbohydrate as compared with a low-fat diet in severe obesity. N Engl J Med 2003;348:2074–2081.

8. Prakash S, Nayyar I, Stern L, Williams M, Chicano K, Daily D, McGrory J, Gracely E, Rader D, Samaha FF. A randomized study comparing the effects of a low-carbohydrate diet and a conventional diet on lipoprotein subfractions and C-reactive protein levels in patients with severe obesity. Am J Med 2004;117:398–405.

9. Sondike SB, Copperman MS, Jacobson MS. Effects of a low-carbohydrate diet on weight loss and cardiovascular risk factor in overweight adolescents. J Pediatr 2003;142:253–258.

10. Ginsberg HN. Hypertriglyceridemia: a risk factor for atherosclerotic cardiovascular disease? A simple question with a complicated answer. Ann Intern Med 1997;126:912–914.

11. Mensink RP, Zock PL, Kester AD, Katan MB. Effects of dietary fatty acids and carbohydrates on the ratio of serum total to HDL cholesterol and on serum lipids and apolipoproteins: a meta-analysis of 60 controlled trials. Am J Clin Nutr 2003;77(5):1146–1155.

12. Meckling KA, O'Sullivan C, Saari D. Comparison of a low-fat diet to a low-carbohydrate diet on weight loss, body composition, and risk factors for diabetes, and cardiovascular disease in free-living, overweight men and women. J Clin Endocrinol Metab 2004;89:2717–2723.

13. Ornish D. Very low-fat diets (correspondence). Circulation 1999;100(9):1013–1014.

14. Nordmann A, Nordmann A, Briel M, Keller U, Yancy W, Brehm B, Bucher H. Effects of low-carbohydrate vs. low-fat diets on weight loss and cardiovascular risk factors. A meta-analysis of randomized controlled trials. Arch Intern Med 2006;166:285–293.

15. Menotti A, Blackburn H, Kromhout D, Nissinen A, Adachi H, Lanti M. Cardiovascular risk factors as determinants of 25-year all cause mortality in the seven countries study. Eur J Epidemiol 2001;17(4);337–346.

16. Sacks F, Castelli W, Donner A, et al. Plasma lipids and lipoproteins in vegetarians and controls. N Engl J Med 1975;292:1148–1151.

17. Pritikin R. The New Pritikin Program: the easy and delicious way to shed fat, lower your cholesterol, and stay fit. New York: Pocket Books, 1991.

18. Ornish D. Eat more, weigh less: Dr. Dean Ornish's Life Choice Program for losing weight safely while eating abundantly. New York: HarperCollins, 2001.

19. Ornish D, Scherwitz, L, Doody, R et al. Effects of stress management training and dietary changes in treating ischemic heart disease. JAMA 1983;249:54–59.

20. Ornish D, Scherwitz L, Billings J, Gould L, Merritt T, Sparler S, Armstrong W, Ports T, Kirkeeide R, Hogeboom C, Brand R. Intensive lifestyle changes for reversal of coronary heart disease. JAMA 1998;280(23):2001–2007.

21. Gould L, Ornish D, Scherwitz L, Brown S, Edens R, Patterson R, Hess M, Mullani N, Bolomey L, Dobbs F, Armstrong W, Merritt T, Ports T, Sparler S, Billings J. Changes in myocardial perfusion abnormalities by positron emission tomography after long-term, intense risk factor modification. JAMA 1995;274(11):894–901.

22. Pirozzo S, Summerbell C, Cameron C, Glasziou P. Advice on low-fat diets for obesity. Cochrane Database Syst Rev 2005;4.

23. Sears B. The Zone: a dietary road map to lose weight permanently: reset your genetic code: prevent disease: achieve maximum physical performance. New York: HarperCollins, 1995.

24. Agatston A. The South Beach Diet: the delicious, doctor-designed, foolproof plan for fast and healthy weight loss. Emmaus, PA: Rodale Press, 2003.

25. Ford ES, Liu S. Glycemic index and serum high-density lipoprotein cholesterol concentration among US adults. Arch Intern Med 2001;26161(4):572–576.

26. Oxlund AL. Glycemic index and glyaecemic load in relation to blood lipids: 6 years of follow-up in adult Danish men and women. Public Health Nutr 2006;9(6):737–745.

27. Aude YW, Agatston AS, Lopez-Jimenez F, Lieberman EH, Marie Almon, Hansen M, Rojas G, Lamas GA, Hennekens CH. The national cholesterol education program diet vs. a diet lower in carbohydrates and higher in protein and monounsaturated fat: a randomial trial. Arch Intern Med 2004;164(19):2141–2146.

28. Dansinger M, Gleason J, Griffith J, Selker H, Schaefer E. Comparison of the Atkins, Ornish, Weight Watchers, and Zone diets for weight loss and heart disease risk reduction. A randomized trial. JAMA 2005;293:43–53.

29. Keyes A. Coronary heart disease in seven countries. Circulation 1970;41(suppl I):1–211.
30. Menotti A, Blackburn H, Kromhout D, Nissinen A, Adachi H, Lanti M. Cardiovascular risk factors as determinants of 25-year all-cause mortality in the seven countries study. Eur J Epidemiol 2001;17(4);337–346.
31. Hu FB. The Mediterranean Diet and mortality: olive oil and beyond. N Engl J Med 2003;348:2595–2596.
32. de Lorgeril M, Salen PT, Martin J, Monjaud I, Delaye J, Mamelle N. Mediterranean diet, traditional risk factors, and the rate of cardiovascular complications after myocardial infarction. Final report of the Lyon Diet Heart Study. Circulation 1999;99:779–785.
33. GISSI–Prevenzione Investigators. Dietary supplementation with n-3 polyunsaturated fatty acids and vitamin E after myocardial infarction: results of the GISSI prevention trial. Gruppo Italiano per lo Studio della Sopravvivenza nell'Infarto miocardico. Lancet 1999;354: 447–455.
34. Barzi F, Woodward M, Marfisi RM, Tavazzi L, Valagussa F, Marchioli R, Gissi-Prevenzine Investigators. Mediterranean diet and all causes mortality after myocardial infarction: results from the GISSI-Prevenzione trial. Eur J Clin Nutr 2003;57(8):1034.
35. Singh R, Dubnov G, Niaz M, Ghosh S, Singh R, Rastogi S, Manor O, Pella D, Berry E. Effect of an Indo-Mediterranean diet on progression of coronary artery disease in high risk patients (Indo-Mediterranean Diet Heart Study): a randomised single-blind trial. Lancet 2002;360:1455–1461.
36. Trichopoulou A, Costacou T, Bamia C, Trichopoulos D. Adherence to a Mediterranean diet and survival in a Greek population. N Engl J Med 2003;348(26):2595–2596.
37. Estruch R, Martinez-Gonzalez M, Corella D, Sala-Salvado J, Ruiz-Gutierrez V, Covas M, Fiol M, Gomez-Gracia E, Lopez-Sabater M, Vinyoles E, Aros F, Conde M, Lahoz C, Lapetr J, Saez G, Ros E, for the PREDIMED Study Investigators. Effects of a Mediterranean-style diet on cardiovascular risk factors. A randomized trial. Ann Intern Med 2006;145:1–11.
38. Lagiou P, Trichopoulos D, Sandin S, Lagiou A, Mucci L, Wolk A, Weiderpass E, Adami HO. Mediterranean dietary pattern and mortality among young women: a cohort study in Sweden. Br J Nutr 2006;96(2):384–392.
39. Knoops K, de Groot L, Kromhout D, Perrin A, Moreiras-Varela O, Menotti A, Staveren W. Mediterranean diet, lifestyle factors, and 10-year mortality in elderly European men and women. The HALE Project. JAMA 2004;292:1433–1439.
40. Pitsavos C, Panagiotakos D, Chrysohoou C, Skoumas J, Papaioannou I, Stefanadis C, Toutouza P. The effect of Mediterranean diet on the risk of the development of acute coronary syndromes in hypercholesterolemic people: a caes-control study (CARDIO 2000). Coron Artery Dis 2002;13:295–300.
41. Bazzano LA, He J, Ogden LG, Loria CM, Vupputuri S, Myers L, Whelton PK. Fruit and vegetable intake and risk of cardiovascular disease in US adults: the first National Health and Nutrition Examination Survey Epidemiologic Follow-up Study. Am J Clin Nutr 2002;76(1):93–99.
42. Psota T, Gebauer S, Kris-Etherton P. Dietary omega-3 fatty acid intake and cardiovascular risk. Am J Cardiol 2006;98(suppl):3i–18i.
43. Esposito K, Marfella R, Ciotola M, Di Palo C, Giugliano F, Giugliano G, D'Armiento M, D'Andrea F, Giugliano D. Effect of a Mediterranean-style diet on endothelial dysfunction and markers of vascular inflammation in the metabolic syndrome: a randomized trial. JAMA 2004;292:1440–1446.
44. Vincent-Baudry S, Defoort C, Gerber M, Bernard M-C, Verger P, Helal O, Portugal H, Planells R, Grolier P, Amiot-Carlin M-J, Vague P, Lairon D. The Medi-RIVAGE study: reduction of cardiovascular disease risk factors after a 3-mo intervention with a Mediterranean-type diet or a low-fat diet. Am J Clin Nutr 2005;82(5):964–971.
45. Chrysohoou C, Panagiotakos DB, Pitsavos C, Das UN, Stefanadis C. Adherence to the Mediterranean diet attenuates inflammation and coagulation process in healthy adults: the ATTICA Study. J Am Coll Cardiol 2004;44(1):152–158.

46. Michalsen A Lehmann N, Pithan C, Knoblauch NT, Moebus S, Kannenberg F, Binder L, Budde T, Dobos GJ. Mediterranean diet has no effect on markers of inflammation and metabolic risk factors in patients with coronary artery disease. Eur J Clin Nutr 2006;60(4):478–485.

47. www.nhlbi.nih.gov/guidelines/cholesterol

48. Lichtenstein A, Appel L, Brands M, Carnethon M, Daniels S, Franch H, Franklin B, Kris-Etherton P, Harris W, Howard B, Karanja N, Lefevre M, Rudel L, Sacks F, Van Horn L, Winston M, Wylie Rosett J. Diet and lifestyle recommendations revision 2006. A scientific statement from the American Heart Association Nutrition Committee. Circulation 2006;114:82–96.

49. Stone N, Nicolosi R, Kris-Etherton P, Ernst N, Krauss R, Winston M. Summary of the scientific conference on the efficacy of hypocholesterolemic dietary interventions. Circulation 1996;94:3388–3391.

50. Yu-Poth S, Guixiang Z, Etherton T, Naglak M, Jonnalagadda S, Kris-Etherton P. Effects of the National Cholesterol Education Program's Step I and Step II dietary intervention programs on cardiovascular disease risk factors: a meta-analysis. Am J Clin Nutr 1999;69: 632–646.

51. Walden CE, Retzlaff BM, Buck BL, McCann BS, Knopp RH. Lipoprotein lipid responses to the National Cholesterol Education Program Step II diet by hypercholesterolemic and combined hyperlipidemic women and men. Arterioscler Thromb Vasc Biol 1997;17(2): 375–382.

52. Flynn MM, Zmuda JM, Milosavljevic D, Caldwell MJ, Herbert PN. Lipoprotein response to a NCEP Step 2 diet with and without energy restriction. Metabolism 1999;48(7):822–826.

53. Walden CE, Retzlaff BM, Buck BL, Wallick S, McCann BS, Knopp RH. Differential effect of NCEP step II diet on HDL cholesterol, its subfractions, and apoprotein A-I levels in hypercholesterolemic women and men after 1 year: the beFIT study. Arterioscler Thromb Vasc Biol 2000;20(6):1580–1587.

54. Wood PD, Stefanick ML, Williams PT, Haskell WL. The effects on plasma lipoproteins of a prudent weight-reducing diet, with or without exercise in overweight men and women. N Engl J Med 1991;325(7):461–466.

55. Stefanick ML, Mackey S, Sheehan M, Ellsworth N, Haskell W, Wood P. Effects of diet and exercise in men and postmenopausal women with low levels of HDL cholesterol and high levels of LDL cholesterol. N Engl J Med 1998;339:12–20.

56. Howard BV, Van Horn L, Hsia J, Manson JE, Stefanick ML, Wassertheil-Smoller S, Kuller LH, LaCroix AZ, Langer RD et al. Low-fat dietary pattern and risk of cardiovascular disease: the Women's Health Initiative Randomized Controlled Dietary Modification Trial. JAMA 2006;295(6):655–666.

57. Hsia J. Rodabough R, Rosal MC, Cochrane B, Howard BV, Snetselaar L, Frishman WH, Stefanick ML. Compliance with National Cholesterol Education Program dietary and lifestyle guidelines among older women with self reported hypercholesterolemia. The Women's Health Initiative. Am J Med 2002;113(5):384–392.

58. Jenkins DJ, Kendall CW, Vidgen E, Mehling CC, Parker T, Seyler H, Faulkner D., Garsetti M, Griffin LC, Agarwal S, Rao AV, Cunnane SC, Ryan MA, Connelly PW, Leiter LA, Vuksan V, Josse R. The effect of serum lipids and oxidized low-density lipoprotein of supplementing self-selected low fat diets with soluble fiber, soy, and vegetable protein. Metabolism 2000;49(1):67–72.

59. Schaefer EJ, Lichenstein AH, Lamon-fava S, Contois JH, Li Z, Goldin BR, Rasmussen H, McNamara JR, Ordovas JM. Effects of NCEP Step 2 diets relatively high or relatively low in fish-derived fatty acids on plasma lipoproteins in middle-aged and elderly subjects. Am J Clin Nutr 1996;63(2):234–241.

60. Bell L, Hectorn K, Reynolds H, Hunninghake D. Cholesterol-lowering effects of soluble-fiber cereals as part of a prudent diet for patients with mild to moderate hypercholesterolemia. Am J Clin Nutr 1990;52;1020–1026.

61. Hu F, Stampfer M, Manson J, Rimm E, Colditz G, Rosner B, Hennekens C, Willett W. Dietary fat intake and the risk of coronary heart disease in women. N Engl J Med 1997;337: 1491–1499.
62. Vega-Lopez S, Ausman LM, Jalbert SM, Erkkila AT, Lichtenstein AH. Palm and partially hydrogenated soybean oils adversely alter lipoprotein profiles compared with soybean and canola oils in moderately hyperlipidemic patients. Am J Clin Nutr 2006;84(1): 54–62.
63. Mensink R, Zock P, Kester A, Katan M. Effects of dietary fatty acids and carbohydrates on the ratio of serum total to HDL cholesterol and on serum lipids and apolipoproteins: a meta analysis of 60 controlled trials. Am J Clin Nutr 2003;77:1146–1155.
64. Joshipura K, Hu FB, Manson J, Stampfer M, Rimm E, Speizer F, Colditz G, Asherio A, Rosner B, Spiegelman D, Willett W. The effect of fruit and vegetable intake on risk for coronary heart disease. Ann Intern Med 2001;134:1106–1114.
65. Hu FB, Rimm EB, Stampfer MJ, Ascherio A, Spiegelman D, Willett WC. Prospective study of major dietary patterns and risk of coronary heart disease. Am J Clin Nutr 2000;72(4): 912–921.
66. Fung TT, Willett WC, Stampfer MJ, Manson JE, Hu FB. Dietary patterns and the risk of coronary heart disease in women. Arch Intern Med 2001;161(15):1857–1862.
67. Steffen LM, Jacobs DR, Stevens J, Shahar E, Carithers T, Folsom AR. Associations of whole-grain, refined-grain, and fruit and vegetable consumption with risks of all-cause mortality and incident coronary artery disease and ischemic stroke: the Atherosclerosis Risk in Communities Study (ARIC). Am J Clin Nutr 2003;78(3):357–358.
68. de Lorgeril, Renaud S, Mamelle N, Salen P, Martin J, Monjaud I, Guidollet J, Touboul P, Delaye J. Mediterranean alpha-linolenic acid rich diet in secondary prevention of coronary heart disease. Lancet 1994;343(8911):1454–1459.
69. Simopoulos AP. The Mediterranean diets: what is so special about the diet of Greece? The scientific evidence. The Center for Genetics, Nutrition, and Health, Washington, DC, USA. J Nutr 2001;131(11 suppl):3065S–3073S.
70. Azadbakht L, Mirmiran P, Esamaillzadeh A, Azizi T, Azizi F. Beneficial effects of a dietary approaches to stop hypertension eating plan on features of the metabolic syndrome. Diabetes Care 2005;28:2823–2831.
71. Lichtenstein A, Appel L, Brands M, Carnethon M, Daniels S, Franch H, Franklin B, Kris-Etherton P, Harris W, Howard B, Karanja N, Lefevre M, Rudel L, Sacks F, Van Horn L, Winston M, Wylie-Rosett J. AHA UPDATE: diet and lifestyle recommendations revision 2006. A scientific statement from the American Heart Association Nutrition Committee. Circulation 2006;114:82–96.

Suggested Key Readings

Dansinger M, Gleason J, Griffith J, Selker H, Schaefer E. Comparison of the Atkins, Ornish, Weight Watchers, and Zone Diets for weight loss and heart disease risk reduction. A randomized trial. JAMA 2005;293:43–53.
de Lorgeril M, Salen PT, Martin J, Monjaud I, Delaye J, Mamelle N. Mediterranean diet, traditional risk factors, and the rate of cardiovascular complications after myocardial infarction. Final report of the Lyon Diet Heart Study. Circulation 1999;99:779–785.
Lichtenstein A, Appel L, Brands M, Carnethon M, Daniels S, Franch H, Franklin B, Kris-Etherton P, Harris W, Howard B, Karanja N, Lefevre M, Rudel L, Sacks F, Van Horn L, Winston M, Wylie-Rosett J. AHA UPDATE: diet and lifestyle recommendations revision 2006. A scientific statement from the American Heart Association Nutrition Committee. Circulation 2006;114:82–96.

Nordmann A, Nordmann A, Briel M, Keller U, Yancy W, Brehm B, Bucher H. Effects of low-carbohydrate vs. low-fat diets on weight loss and cardiovascular risk factors. A meta-analysis of randomized controlled trials. Arch Intern Med 2006;166:285–293.

Ornish D, Scherwitz L, Billings J, Gould L, Merritt T, Sparler S, Armstrong W, Ports T, Kirkeeide R, Hogeboom C, Brand R. Intensive lifestyle changes for reversal of coronary heart disease. JAMA 1998;280(23);2001–2007.

Chapter 4
Therapeutic Foods

Sarah Sallee Jones

Introduction

The National Cholesterol Education Program Adult Treatment Panel III (NCEP/ATP III) recommends Therapeutic Lifestyle Changes as the cornerstone of treatment for dyslipidemia in all patients. In addition to diets for weight loss and weight maintenance, many patients can benefit from the addition of foods and supplements that directly lower serum cholesterol. In fact, many patients prefer the use of therapeutic foods over the use of pharmacologic agents because they see this as a more natural form of therapy.

It is crucial that physicians are informed about the broad range of therapeutic foods available as well as what evidence exists for the benefits or harms attributed to certain foods and supplements. This chapter explores many of the foods and supplements that are currently consumed by our patients to help control their cholesterol levels and reduce their cardiac risk. Foods that have more and generally beneficial effects are reviewed *first*; foods with less available evidence or information are reviewed toward the *end* of the chapter. This chapter should serve as a useful guide for primary care physicians to aid their patients in making wise dietary choices regarding cardiovascular benefit.

Plant Sterols and Stanols

Plant sterols and stanols are naturally occurring substances that structurally resemble cholesterol and are essential components of plant cell membranes. Plant sterols are present in small quantities in many fruits, vegetables, nuts, seeds, legumes and other plant sources, and cereals. Plant stanols, the saturated counterparts of plant sterols, occur naturally in even smaller quantities from some of the same sources. Both plant

S.S. Jones
Associate Program Director, Family Medicine Residency, Department of Family Medicine, David Grant Medical Center, Travis Air Force Base, CA

B.V. Reamy (ed.), *Hyperlipidemia Management for Primary Care*,
DOI: 10.1007/978-0-387-76606-5_4, © Springer Science+Business Media, LLC 2008

sterols and stanols are also found in vegetable oils, especially soybean oil. They have been recognized to have cholesterol-lowering effects, when consumed in sufficient amounts, since the 1950s [1].

Plant sterols and stanols displace exogenous cholesterol in the intestinal lumen, thus lowering serum cholesterol by decreasing its absorption by intestinal transport proteins (ABCG5, ABCG8, NPC1L1) [2]. They may also influence cellular cholesterol metabolism within intestinal enterocytes [3] and subsequently increase endogenous cholesterol synthesis. Plant sterols and stanols do not appear to have a significant effect on serum triglyceride or high density lipoprotein cholesterol (HDL-C) levels.

The esterified forms of plant sterols and stanols have been incorporated into food products that are directly available to consumers in grocery stores. The first products to gain popularity were in the form of margarines and spreads, such as Benecol® and Take Control®. Other products are now available, including Minute Maid® HeartWise® orange juice, Yoplait® Healthy Heart yogurt, Rice Dream® HeartWise® rice milk, Nature Valley® Healthy Heart granola bars, Oroweat® Whole Grain Oat Bread, and Lifetime® Low Fat Cheese (formulated with CoroWise™ Phytosterols Esters). These products appear to be equally efficacious in lowering total and low density lipoprotein cholesterol (LDL-C) compared to placebo [3–8]. Multiple studies have shown a cholesterol-lowering effect of as much as 15% when sufficient amounts of these products are consumed; maximum benefit is achieved at doses of 2–3 g per day [9–14].

There has been a concern that consumption of plant sterols and stanols may potentially lower serum fat-soluble vitamins such as A, D, and E. Although some studies have shown transient decreases in levels of beta-carotene [15], there is no evidence that any clinically significant reduction in serum vitamin levels results from plant sterol or stanol esters [16–18].

The cholesterol-lowering benefit of plant sterols and stanols appears to cross many subgroups of individuals with hypercholesterolemia. These substances appear to be safe and effective in both diabetics and nondiabetics [19], in children and adults with familial hypercholesterolemia [20–22], and in patients with mild to moderate hypercholesterolemia [4,7,16,18]. Multiple short-term studies show a similar cholesterol-lowering effect with both plant stanol and plant sterol ester spreads, but some studies have suggested that the cholesterol-lowering benefit of plant stanols may be more sustainable than with plant sterols [23,24]. More studies are needed to determine whether plant stanol-fortified foods should be chosen over plant sterol-fortified foods.

Combination Therapy

Plant sterol and stanol esters are a potential adjunct to statin therapy for patients with hypercholesterolemia who have not met their target LDL-C goal with diet and statin therapy [25–27]. A meta-analysis of 41 trials found an additive effect with a combination of dietary intervention, statin therapy, and plant stanols or sterols.

The authors reported that adding sterols or stanols to statins lowers cholesterol more effectively than doubling the statin dose [28].

There does not appear to be an additive effect with the combination of plant sterols and ezetimibe, which also exerts its cholesterol-lowering effect by decreased intestinal cholesterol absorption. Used alone, 10 mg daily of ezetimibe lowered LDL-C significantly more than 2 g/day of plant sterols (22% versus 4.7%) [29–31].

Recommendations: Based on the results of multiple studies and meta-analyses, several organizations have made formal recommendations regarding the therapeutic effect of plant stanols and sterols on lowering serum cholesterol levels. The National Cholesterol Education Program Adult Treatment Panel III (NCEP/ATP III) Report asserted that the use of plant stanols/sterols in bioavailable forms should be a "key element" of maximal dietary therapy [30]. Recent studies of plant sterol and stanol esters in humans have shown that maximum cholesterol-lowering benefits are achieved at doses of 2-3 g per day [9–14]. Intakes greater than this amount do not seem to yield any additional cholesterol reductions and are thus not recommended [27]. A study published in the *Journal of the American Dietetic Association* found that only 2-3 patients (2.8 pts) would need to be treated with the 2 g/day plant sterol/stanol prescription to obtain a reduction in cholesterol by ≥15 percent compared with dietary changes alone [31].

AHA Recommendations: In 2006, the American Heart Association Nutrition Committee supported consumption (up to 2 grams daily for maximal benefit) of plant stanols/sterols by individuals with elevated LDL cholesterol, in addition to diet and lifestyle modification, as a therapeutic option for lowering LDL cholesterol [14]. It is not clear whether plant sterols/stanol esters should be used in individuals with normal cholesterol levels who have other risk factors for coronary artery disease. When used in hypercholesterolemic children, it is prudent to monitor fat-soluble vitamin status.

Omega-3 Polyunsaturated Fatty Acids (PUFAs)

Fish oil has long been associated with health benefits. Societies that naturally consume large amounts of fish, particularly oily fish, have lower rates of cardiovascular disease. Interest in omega-3 fatty acids was heightened in the 1970s when low rates of coronary events in Greenland Eskimos who consumed large amounts of fish and seal in their diets were demonstrated [1].

Omega-3 fatty acids, in particular, eicosapentaenoic acid (EPA) and docosahexaenoic acid (DHA), have been shown to have antiinflammatory, antiarrhythmic, and antilipemic effects. EPA and DHA are primarily obtained from fatty fish, such as mackerel, salmon, herring, anchovy, sardines, and lake trout. EPA and DHA are also converted from the intermediate-chain α-linolenic acid, which is found in canola, soybean, flaxseed, and walnut oils, nuts, and vegetables of the cabbage family [1].

Studies of Cardiac Outcomes and Mortality

Several large studies and numerous small studies have shown that omega-3 fatty acids reduce sudden cardiac death and total mortality.

Gruppo Italiano per lo Studio della Sopravvivenza nell'Infarto Miocardico (GISSI)

The Gruppo Italiano per lo Studio della Sopravvivenza nell'Infarto Miocardico (GISSI)-Prevenzione trial is the largest secondary prevention study on fatty acids to date. The GISSI trial evaluated the effect of fish oil therapy on 11,234 patients who had a myocardial infarction in the 3 months before enrollment. In addition to consuming a heart-healthy Mediterranean diet and concomitant therapy with aspirin, statins, and/or beta-blockers, patients were randomized to receive fish oil (1 capsule, EPA + DHA), vitamin E 300 mg/day, both fish oil and vitamin E, or standard care alone for a mean duration of 3.5 years. Primary endpoints—death, nonfatal myocardial infarction (MI), and stroke—were reduced by 15% with fish oil treatment; vitamin E had no effect on any endpoint [32]. Secondary endpoints revealed a 45% reduction in sudden death and 21% decrease in total mortality. Thus, the cardioprotective effects were additive to diet and to standard pharmacotherapy [33]. A subgroup analysis of the GISSI trial findings attributed the reduction in sudden death through an antiarrhythmogenic effect. The benefit of omega-3 fatty acids on sudden cardiac death increased proportionately in individuals with progressively worse left ventricular systolic function [34].

The Indian Study on Infarct Survival (ISIS)

The Indian Study on Infarct Survival (ISIS) [35] included 360 postinfarction patients. It demonstrated a 30% reduction in total cardiac events, including sudden cardiac death, total cardiac deaths, and nonfatal reinfarction, in patients who were randomized to receive fish oil within 24 h following an MI versus patients randomized to receive mustard seed oil or placebo. This study is unique compared to other studies, as patients were enrolled within 24 h of having an MI, and the majority did not receive typical postinfarction therapies such as beta-blockers (only 30% of patients) or angiotensin-converting enzyme inhibitors (20% of patients).

The Japan EPA Lipid Study (JELIS)

The Japan EPA Lipid Intervention Study (JELIS) [36] is a large primary and secondary prevention trial that randomized 14,981 patients for primary prevention and 3,664 patients for secondary prevention. The study was a prospective open-label blinded endpoint study with a 4.6-year follow-up. Patients consumed their typical diet rich in omega-3 fatty acids and were given low-dose statin therapy. The incidence of major coronary events, including nonfatal MI, coronary artery disease (CAD) death, unstable angina, and revascularization procedures, were reduced 19% at the end of the study period. The incidence of unstable angina and nonfatal coronary events was significantly reduced, but there was no change in the incidence of sudden death and coronary death. LDL and HDL levels did not change significantly after treatment. Changes in the serum ratio of omega-3 fatty acids to omega-6 fatty acids were predictive of coronary death and MI. These findings suggest that in populations consuming large quantities of fish, higher doses of omega-3 fatty acids confer cardioprotective effects by other mechanisms, including plaque stabilization [37].

The Diet and Reinfarction Trial (DART)

The Diet and Reinfarction Trial (DART) [38] was a randomized, factorial-design intervention trial of 2033 men with recent MI. Subjects were randomized to receive or not receive dietary advice that included reduced fat intake, increased consumption of cereal fiber, and increased fatty fish intake (two fatty fish meals/week). Study endpoints included total mortality, death from ischemic heart disease, and nonfatal MI. After 2 years of follow-up, those advised to eat fatty fish had a 29% decline in mortality. There was a slightly increased incidence in nonfatal events, indicating that patients survived MIs that would have otherwise been fatal.

The Physicians' Health Study

The Physicians' Health Study demonstrated that men who consumed nuts two or more times per week had significant reductions in total coronary deaths and sudden cardiac deaths (relative risk, 0.53 and 0.70, respectively) compared to men who rarely or never consumed nuts [39].

Meta-Analyses

Other studies have demonstrated that omega-3 fish oil therapy is additive to diet and standard pharmacotherapy with statins, beta-blockers, and aspirin. A meta-analysis of nine secondary prevention studies [40] involving more than 9200 patients demonstrated a similar reduction in total mortality to that seen in patients treated with statin therapy (20% versus 22% reduction). A meta-analysis of 11 placebo- or diet-controlled trials of omega-3 fatty acid therapy found a significant 20% reduction in total mortality after 6 months or more of therapy. Five of these studies enrolled patients with established coronary artery disease [41].

Conflicting Studies

Not all secondary prevention studies have demonstrated a significant reduction in morbidity and mortality in post-MI patients treated with omega-3 fatty acids. In Nilsen's study of 300 Norwegian patients treated with omega-3 fatty acids or a corn oil placebo within 1 week of an MI, no clinical benefit from fish oil was demonstrated regarding cardiac death, cardiac resuscitation, recurrent MI, or unstable angina [42]. The patients enrolled in the study consumed a baseline diet of fish with a high omega-3 fatty acid content; observational studies suggest that there may be a threshold for omega-3 fatty acid of 5.5 g/month (96 g/week of fish), above which there is not a mortality benefit [43]. Also, corn oil itself contains linoleic acid, which may have antiarrhythmic properties [44].

In a recent systematic review involving 48 randomized controlled trials (RCTs) and 41 observational studies of 30,000 patients, omega-3 supplementation did not significantly reduce mortality or the likelihood of a cardiovascular event [45]. These findings conflict with the GISSI and JELIS studies, which also had approximately 30,000 enrollees.

Studies of Antiarrhythmic Effects

The effects of omega-3 fatty acids have been studied in several large randomized trials. Calo et al. conducted a study of 160 patients who were undergoing elective bypass surgery [46]. Patients were randomized to treatment with omega-3 fatty acids 5 days before surgery through the time of hospital discharge. The patients were followed for 1 month after discharge to assess the incidence of postoperative atrial fibrillation. Omega-3 fatty acid therapy given perioperatively was found to be a significant independent predictor of postoperative atrial fibrillation at 1 month, with 15.2% of patients who received omega-3 fatty acids affected versus 33.3% of patients who received usual care.

The Study on Omega-3 Fatty Acid and Ventricular Arrhythmia (SOFA)

The Study on Omega-3 Fatty Acid and Ventricular Arrhythmia (SOFA) was a randomized, double-blind, multicenter trial conducted in Europe investigating the antiarrhythmic effects of omega-3 fatty acids on the primary endpoint of recurrent spontaneous ventricular tachycardia or fibrillation and all-cause mortality [47]. In this study, 546 patients with an implantable cardiac defibrillator (ICD) in place and at least one episode of ventricular tachycardia or fibrillation during the previous year were enrolled; 63% of the enrollees had a recent MI, and 55% had baseline ventricular tachycardia. Patients were randomized to receive a supplement of fish oil versus placebo of high oleic acid sunflower oil for 12 months. In contrast to the JELIS study already described, patients were excluded if they typically consumed a high or moderate amount of fish in their diets or used fish oil supplements during the 3 months before screening. At 1 year, there was no significant difference in event-free survival between the two groups, including a subgroup analysis of patients with prior MI. A negative effect of fish oil therapy was not seen in any subgroup of patients.

The Fatty Acid Antiarrhythmia Trial (FAAT)

The Fatty Acid Antiarrhythmia Trial (FAAT) was a randomized double-blind study conducted in the United States [48]. This 12-month study evaluated the effects of omega-3 fatty acids versus olive oil placebo in 402 patients with ICDs placed for history of cardiac arrest, history of sustained ventricular tachycardia, or sustained ventricular tachycardia or fibrillation during electrophysiological studies. At the end of the study, 28% of patients who received fish oil reached the primary endpoint of ventricular tachycardia, ventricular fibrillation, or death compared with 39% of patients in the control group, representing a 28% risk reduction in the treatment group. Notably, compliance was problematic in this study; by the end of the study, 35% of patients in both treatment groups discontinued their prescribed supplements. After adjusting for study participants who complied with their assigned regimen for at least 11 months, the risk reduction approached 38%.

Raitt and colleagues performed a study of 200 patients with a history of ventricular tachycardia or fibrillation who subsequently had implantable cardiac defibrillators (ICDs) placed [49]. Patients were excluded if they were taking class I or class III antiarrhythmic agents or if they had episodes of sustained ventricular tachycardia or fibrillation outside the setting of acute MI. Of the patients, 55% had a prior, but not recent, MI; 66% of enrollees had baseline ventricular tachycardia. Patients were randomized to treatment with 1.8 g/day omega-3 fatty acid supplements or an olive oil placebo for 2 years. The primary endpoint was time to first episode of ICD treatment for ventricular tachycardia or fibrillation. There was a trend toward an increased incidence of ventricular tachycardia and fibrillation observed in the treatment group, suggesting that the supplements may have had proarrhythmic effects in the patients enrolled in their study. One possible explanation for the study's results is that many of the patients may have had scar-based reentry arrhythmia not amenable to antiarrhythmic therapy [37]. The results of this study also raise the possibility that the reduction in sudden cardiac death observed in the GISSI trial may be most pronounced in the setting of acute ischemia or recent MI; alternatively, the reduction in cardiac deaths may not have been caused by suppression of ventricular tachycardia or fibrillation [1].

Patients with Implantable Cardiac Defibrillators (ICDs)

In patients with ICDs, studies of omega-3 fatty acid supplementation have not definitively demonstrated benefit in reducing the risk of CAD mortality or reducing the incidence of ventricular arrhythmias, although there is a trend toward favorable effects in certain subpopulations. One of the proposed mechanisms for the antiarrhythmic effect of omega-3 fatty acids is via correction of defective ion transport from sodium pump failure; thus, ischemia-driven (versus scar-based) arrhythmias are likely to be more responsive to the effects of omega-3 fatty acids [50].

Studies of Lipid-Lowering Effects

In addition to the large studies already cited hallmarking the antiarrhythmic effects and effects on mortality of fatty acids, fatty acids are effective for treating hypertriglyceridemia, an independent risk factor for coronary heart disease [51]. A meta-analysis showed that fish oil, at 2–4 g/day, reduces serum triglyceride levels by 25% to 34% and increases LDL 5% to 10% and HDL levels by 1% to 3% [51].

Multiple organizations have made official statements regarding omega-3 fatty acid intake. The United States Food and Drug Administration has found consumption of EPA + DHA to be safe so long as it does not exceed 3 g/person/day. Supplements containing EPA + DHA are not federally regulated [52].

Nuts

Walnuts, almonds, and macadamia nuts favorably affect serum lipids. Small studies have demonstrated that total cholesterol, LDL-C, and triglycerides are lowered in healthy and hyperlipidemic individuals who consume these nuts [53–56].

AHA Recommendations: In 2002, the American Heart Association made the following recommendations for omega-3 fatty acid intake [54]. For primary prevention, i.e., patients with no known history of coronary heart disease (CHD), intake of a variety of fish (preferably oily) at least twice/week (400-500 mg/week of EPA + DHA) is recommended. Individuals are also advised to include oils and food rich in alpha-linolenic acid. Patients with documented CHD (secondary prevention) are advised to consume 1 g EPA + DHA daily, preferably from oily fish. Capsule supplements may be used in consultation with a physician. Patients with hypertriglyceridemia (>500 mg/dl) are advised to consume 2-4 g/day EPA+DHA in capsules in consultation with a physician (Table 4.1). Similarly, the World Health Organization and many countries have set forth population-based dietary recommendations for fatty acid intake. Most generally advise a range of 300-600 mg EPA+DHA daily [55].

Fish Oil Supplements: Most fish oil capsules available over-the-counter (OTC) in the United States contain approximately 300 mg DHA plus EHA. They can be taken at any time of the day with or without food, together or in divided doses. Although typically well-tolerated, some people experience a "fishy burp," which may be eliminated by taking the capsules at bedtime, freezing them, taking enteric-coated capsules, or taking them with food [56]. Other patients complain of "fishy sweat": this can be lessened by allowing at least 4 hours between vigorous exercise and fish oil ingestion.

Table 4.1 Summary recommendations of therapeutic foods and supplements associated with lipid-lowering effects

Therapeutic food or Supplement	Sources	Evidence	Effects	Recommendation
Plant sterols or stanols	Several forms available in grocery stores	Multiple RCTs	4%–8% TC reduction; 10%–14% LDL reduction	2–3 g/day
Omega-3 fatty acids	Oily fish, DHA + EPA supplements, Omacor® tablets	Multiple RCTs and meta-analyses	Improved morbidity and mortality s/p MI; potentially antiarrhythmic; lowers TG 25%–34%	See Table 4.2
Soluble fiber	Oatmeal, barley, pears, legumes, psyllium	Multiple RCTs and meta-analyses	4% TC reduction; 7%–12% LDL reduction	3–10 g/day
Chocolate	Dark chocolate/ cocoa (rich sources of flavonoids)	Small RCTs and meta-analyses	Mortality decreased; 10%–12% LDL reduction; 4%–13% HDL increase	50–100 g/day; more studies are needed to establish dosage
Alcohol	Red wine (excellent source of the flavonoid resveratrol)	Multiple studies and meta-analysis	HDL increased; LDL oxidation inhibited; mortality decreased	5 oz/day
Went yeast	Cholestin®	Small studies	16% TC reduction; 22% LDL reduction; 11% TG reduction	2.4 g/day; more studies are needed
Soy protein	Tofu, tempeh, miso, soymilk, soybeans/nuts; soy pills, and extracts/ isoflavones are not recommended	Multiple RCTs and meta-analyses	5%–6% LDL reduction; 7% TG reduction	25 g/day; may be useful as a substitute for animal and dairy products that contain saturated fat and cholesterol

Table 4.1 (continued)

Therapeutic food or Supplement	Sources	Evidence	Effects	Recommendation
Artichoke leaf extract	OTC supplement	Small RCTs	18.5% TC reduction; 23% LDL reduction	1800 mg/day; larger, quality studies are needed to establish definitive role
Garlic	Fresh garlic; garlic tablets; garlic powder; garlic oil	Multiple RCTs and meta-analyses	Mixed results of lipid-lowering effect	Supplements not recommended; 1–2 cloves/day fresh garlic for culinary use
Folic acid	OTC (or prescription) supplement	Multiple studies	Reduces homo-cysteine levels; no beneficial effect on cardiovas-cular mortality or lipid levels	Not recommended for cardiovascular benefit
Vitamin E	Vitamin E	Multiple RCTs and meta-analyses	High dose (400 IU/day or more) associated with increased mortality; no effect on lipid levels	Not recommended for cardiovascular benefit
Fenugreek	Plant/potherb	Small studies	Increased HDL; decreased TG and total cholesterol	5–30 g/day defatted fenugreek vs. 1 g/day fenugreek extract; larger, quality studies are needed to establish definitive role
Coenzyme Q10	OTC supplement	Multiple small studies	Small increase in HDL; small reduction in lipoprotein a and TG	120–150 mg/day; larger studies are needed to establish definitive role
Myrrh	Herbal extracts	Small studies	4%–5% LDL increase	Not recommended at this time

Table 4.1 (continued)

Therapeutic food or Supplement	Sources	Evidence	Effects	Recommendation
Eggplant	OTC supplement	Small studies	No significant difference in lipid levels	Not recommended at this time
Holy basil	Herbal extract	Few small studies	Possible lipid (and glycemic)-lowering effect	Insufficient evidence to recommend at this time; more studies needed

RCT, randomized controlled trial; TG, triglycerides; MI, myocardial infarction; LDH, low density lipoprotein; HDL, high density lipoprotein; OCT, over the counter.

Table 4.2 American Heart Association (AHA) recommendations for omega-3 fatty acid intake

Patient population	AHA recommendation
Hypertriglyceridemia	Consume 2–4 g/day EPA plus DHA in capsules (in consultation with a physician)
History of coronary heart disease	Consume 1 g/day EPA plus DHA; preferable source: oily fish; supplements may also be used in consultation with a physician
No known history of coronary heart disease	Eat a variety of fish at least twice a week, preferably oily fish; include oils and foods rich in α-linolenic acid

EPA, eicosapentaenoic acid; DHA, docosahexaenoic acid

Source: Adapted with permission from Kris-Etherton PM, Harris WS, Appel LJ, for the Nutrition Committee. Fish consumption, fish oil, omega-3 fatty acids, and cardiovascular disease. Circulation 2002;106:2747–2757 [53].

Omacor® is a new prescription form of highly concentrated fish oil that contains 850 mg EPA + DHA. Due to a unique manufacturing process, it may cause less side effects than over-the-counter fish oil. Four 1-g capsules /day are indicated for treating severe hypertriglyceridemia and are the equivalent of 12 OTC fish oil capsules [57].

Summary: The large secondary prevention trials demonstrate that patients with coronary artery disease who do not typically consume high quantities of fish in their diets will experience a 20 percent reduction in total mortality and cardiovascular deaths when supplemented with low-dose (1 g/day) supplementation of omega-3 fatty acids. Patients who consume large amounts of fish in their diets, such as those enrolled in the JELIS trial, appear to benefit from the plaque-stabilizing property of omega-3 fatty acids, with observed reductions in unstable angina and nonfatal events, but not in sudden or cardiac death [37]. The results of the ICD studies suggest a possible reduction in arrhythmias in some populations. It is too early to determine whether fish oil supplementation should be implemented immediately after MI; the results of ISIS may prompt further study in this arena. No significant side effects were reported in any of the studies. Factors that may affect omega-3 fatty acids' effects on outcomes include: dose and source of omega-3 fatty acids administered (supplements, diet, or both), background diet composition, and duration or treatment, as well as risk level of patients enrolled [37]. Fish oil supplementation can directly reduce serum triglyceride levels and can be used as an adjunct to other lipid lowering medications for this purpose.

Chocolate

Chocolate has long been used as a medicinal remedy and has gained interest in today's health circles because of its antioxidant potential. It contains flavonoids, which are polyphenolic compounds from plants with antioxidant effects. They are hypothesized to provide cardioprotective effects because of their ability to scavenge free radicals and inhibit lipid oxidation. Chocolate also contains the saturated fatty acid (SFA) stearic acid. Saturated fat has long been thought to contribute to atherosclerosis, but stearic acid may be nonatherogenic and noncholesterolemic [57–59].

Several small studies have shown that consuming dark chocolate delays LDL oxidation, reducing serum LDL levels by 10% to 12% [60,61]. Dark chocolate and cocoa consumption appears to have variable effects on HDL-C levels, with several studies reporting a mild to moderate increase of 4% to 13% [58,59,61] and other studies demonstrating no significant change [60].

Flavonoids

Flavonoids are a class of antioxidants derived from plant polyphenols. They are thought to be protective against cardiovascular disease by a number of different mechanisms: antioxidant, antiplatelet, and antiinflammatory effects, increasing HDL, lowering blood pressure, and improving endothelial function by increasing local production of nitric acid by chocolate flavonoids [62]. Flavonoids inhibit LDL oxidation [59,62,63] via their ability to scavenge free radicals and reduce thrombotic tendency in vitro [62,63]. Cocoa polyphenols have been shown to have antiinflammatory effects on the lipoxygenase pathway and to modulate production of inflammatory markers such as interleukin-2. Flavonoids are subdivided into flavones, flavonols, flavanols, and other anthocyanins. Flavanols are further subdived into catechins, epicatechins, procyanidins, and prodelphinidins. Catechins and epicate-chin have antiplatelet effects similar to aspirin [62].

Sources of Flavonoids

Flavonoids are found in teas, apples, onions, and red wine, but cocoa contains greater amounts of flavonoids per serving than all teas and red wines [60,62]. Dark chocolate contains substantially higher amounts of flavonoids, polyphenols, and catechins than milk chocolate; levels of epicatechin in dark chocolate are compa-rable to red wine and tea. The biological effects of flavonoids may be greater in dark chocolate because the intestinal absorption of flavonoids may be inhibited by the milk in milk chocolate [62].

Studies

Prospective studies of flavonoids suggest that flavonoid intake is associated with lower rates of coronary heart disease mortality and lower risk of myocardial infrac-tion. Most studies indicate no association for risk of stroke, although these were small studies with insufficient power. The results of the meta-analysis indicate a significant protective association between flavonoid intake and risk of coronary heart disease (CHD) mortality [relative risk (RR) = 0.81; 95% confidence interval (CI), 0.71–0.92] [62].

Stearic Acid

Stearic acid is a long-chain SFA found commonly in meats and dairy products. Cocoa butter, a fat derived from cocoa plants and found predominantly in dark chocolate, contains an average of 33% oleic acid, 25% palmitic acid, and 33% stearic acid. A meta-analysis of 60 controlled feeding trials concluded that stearic acid neither lowers HDL nor increases LDL or total cholesterol [64]. There are several proposed mechanisms to explain how stearic acid may be cholesterol neutral, but the exact mechanism is not known [62].

Studies

Several studies have explored the association between stearic acid and flavonoids and cardiovascular outcomes. A meta-analysis of 136 experimental, observational, and clinical studies of the relationships between the stearic acid and flavonoids found in cocoa and chocolate and the risk of cardiovascular disease (CVD) has also been performed. This meta-analysis concluded that stearic acid has a neutral effect on cardiovascular disease [62] and that no epidemiologic study to date has appropriately answered the causal question of the association of dietary stearic acid intake and risk of CVD. Flavonoids, on the other hand, are likely protective against CVD [62].

Summary: There is no well-established recommended dose of chocolate, although one author suggests eating 50 g of dark chocolate per day [65]. Another study demonstrated a significant increase in HDL-C with dark chocolate consumption of 75 g/day [61]. Long-term randomized feeding trials are warranted to more definitively determine the long-term impact of chocolate on cardiovascular outcomes, as well as to establish the recommended daily dose to achieve beneficial effects. Consumption of dark chocolate and cocoa powder for their antioxidant benefits should be incorporated into a heart healthy diet that includes other sources of antioxidants such as fruits, vegetables, fish, tea, and wine.

Soluble Fiber

Soluble fiber, a bile acid sequestrant, is associated with cholesterol reduction. It is readily obtained through a variety of food sources, including fruits, vegetables, cereals, and legumes. The U.S. Food and Drug Administration states that four servings per day of two dietary fibers, beta-glucan (0.75 g/serving) and psyllium (1.78 g/serving), would lower cardiovascular disease risk [65,66]. Beta-glucan is found in barley and oatmeal; psyllium is found in Metamucil®. Other forms of soluble fiber include pectins, gums, oat bran, beans, and pears. An excellent source of information regarding the soluble fiber content of foods can be found at the National Heart Lung and Blood Institute website: www.nhlbi.nih.gov/chd/Tipsheets/solfiber.htm. Insoluble fiber includes hemicellulose, cellulose, methylcellulose, and lignins [67].

Studies

Jenkins et al. performed an RCT of 68 hyperlipidemic adults who were already on a low-fat, low-cholesterol diet and compared fasting lipids between groups adhering to diet alone versus diet supplemented with four servings/day of foods containing beta-glucan or psyllium [65]. The patients who consumed a high-fiber diet had a total cholesterol level that was reduced modestly (2.1%); total:HDL and LDL:HDL ratios were also reduced 2.9% and 2.4%, respectively. Applying the Framingham cardiovascular disease risk equation to the data resulted in a risk reduction of 4.2% ± 1.4% [66].

One meta-analysis that included eight controlled trials associated the intake of 3 g/day of soluble fiber with a 5 mg/dl reduction in total cholesterol and LDL levels [67]. Another meta-analysis supports this finding [68]. HDL-C and triglyceride levels are not affected by soluble fiber intake [68–76].

> **Dietary Recommendations:** When added to a cholesterol-lowering diet, soluble fiber appears to have modest additive effects in lowering serum cholesterol in both adults and children with mild to moderate hypercholesterolemia [67,70–74]. The recommended, practical intake is 3 g/day of soluble fiber or 3 to 4 servings of soluble fiber rich foods per day. In addition, there may be an additive effect between soluble fiber and treatment with statins; Moreyra et al. showed a similar lowering of LDL-C inpatients who received 20 mg simvastatin and patients who received 10 mg simvastatin plus 15 g psyllium/day [75]. Aller et al. demonstrated that an average daily intake of 3.5 g/day soluble fiber resulted in a 12.8 percent reduction in LDL-C, while other studies have shown a more modest reduction [69,76]. In patients without hypercholesterolemia (loosely defined in one study as a total cholesterol <240 mg/dl), there was no statistically significant reduction seen in total, LDL, or HDL cholesterol after 3 months of treatment with 8 g/day of soluble fiber [77].

Red Wine and Alcohol

Excessive alcohol intake is a significant public health problem in the United States. Current estimates are that 10% of Americans suffer with some form of an alcohol abuse disorder. Overconsumption of alcohol is responsible for several deleterious health outcomes, including hypertension, increased body mass index (BMI), cirrhosis, bone marrow suppression, suicides, and violent death—especially from motor vehicle trauma.

Against this backdrop of concern with overuse of alcohol, a steady stream of research studies have confirmed the health benefits of a low to moderate level of alcohol consumption for reducing cardiovascular clinical outcomes and increasing longevity. There is a strong inverse relationship between ethanol intake and the occurrence of myocardial infarction and cardiac death [77,78].

The "French Paradox," or the concept that reduced rates of cardiovascular disease in France seem to be related to an increase in daily red wine consumption, also added to interest in research about specific forms of alcohol that are ingested and whether different forms have increased health benefits [79].

Dose

All the studies that have suggested a health benefit from low or moderate consumption of alcohol have demonstrated this benefit at the equivalent of *less than* three drinks per day. One drink per day appears more beneficial for women, and two for men. A drink is defined as 5 oz wine, 1 oz liquor, or 12 oz beer (with 6% ethanol). Consumption of alcohol above these levels is associated with a steady increase in negative health outcomes. In fact, there is a definite J-shaped curve relating alcohol or wine intake to mortality. Mortality is lowest for moderate drinkers and increases for nondrinkers or for heavy drinkers [80–82].

Wine

Mortality is even lower for wine drinkers than for drinkers of other forms of alcohol [81]. The initial project demonstrating this was done by St. Leger, who studied variables associated with cardiovascular death in 18 countries. He found a strong and specific inverse relationship between cardiac deaths and alcohol consum-ption; this association seemed to be entirely because of wine consumption [83]. Several more studies have confirmed this early observation that, of consumers of alcohol, those who consume red wine have the greatest health benefits.

In one of the most definitive meta-analyses, Groenback et al. examined the relationship of consuming different forms of alcohol, death from all causes, and CHD death. They pooled data from three studies and more than 13,000 men and 22,000 women. At all levels of alcohol intake, wine drinkers were at a significantly lower risk than non-wine drinkers for all-cause mortality and CHD death (P less than 0.001) [84].

Biological Mechanisms: Alcohol and Resveratrol

Alcohol has several beneficial biological effects that help to protect against cardiovascular disease. Foremost is the ability of alcohol to directly increase HDL. At present, alcohol is one of the most potent inducers of HDL increase [85]. In addition, alcohol directly reduces platelet reactivity and aggregation [85]. It will also prolong bleeding times.

Wine has health benefits above those that can be attributed just to its alcohol content. Red wine in particular is a rich source of flavonoids. Chief among them is resveratrol. Resveratrol is a phenolic compound that gives wine many of its sensory and gustatory properties, and it has been investigated by chemists for decades. Resveratrol is derived from the grape skin and is found chiefly in red wine, which spends a long time in contact with grape skin as compared to white wine, which spends minimal grape skin contact time.

Resveratrol is a potent antioxidant and is responsible for slowing the aging of red wine. Moderate red wine consumption directly increases plasma antioxidant activity and inhibits the oxidation of LDL cholesterol and improves endothelial function; this directly inhibits the formation of atherosclerotic plaque [86]. Resveratrol also has antiinflammatory effects and inhibits the activity of monocytes and macrophage accumulation at areas of intimal damage, which provides additional antiatherosclerotic effects on the endothelium.

Red Grape Juice

Resveratrol is also present in pure red grape juice but at levels approximately nine times lower than in red wine. Red grape juice has also been shown to have antioxidant properties in vitro. For patients who do not want to drink alcohol, red grape juice is a useful adjunct for reducing cardiovascular risk. However, it would require an intake of 45 oz per day of red grape juice to equal the antioxidant amounts in a single 5-oz glass of red wine.

Summary: Alcohol consumed in moderation reduces the risk of coronary events and death. Red wine has additional protective effects above and beyond those attributed to alcohol. These are felt to be secondary to the anti-oxidant and anti-atherogenic properties of resveratrol, which is a flavonoid present at high concentrations in red wine. Given the significant health risks of alcohol abuse in the United States, physicians should recommend alcohol to patients in the same way they dispense prescription medications. It should be done prudently and on an individual basis, taking into account the health status of the patient as well as their cultural preferences regarding the consumption of alcohol.

Soy Protein

Soy protein is an edible component of the soybean, *Glycine max*. Soy protein is produced from raw whole soybeans by a multistep process that removes the lipid and indigestible components to concentrate the protein and increase its availability. Depending on the particular steps used during processing, soy protein ingredients may take the form of isolated soy protein (ISP), soy protein concentrate, or soy flour. Each ingredient may be further processed into texturized soy protein or texturized vegetable protein (TVP). In addition to protein, these soy protein ingredients contain other naturally occurring soy constituents, such as isoflavones, fiber, and saponins [87]. Soy protein contains all the essential amino acids in sufficient quantities to support human life and is therefore a complete protein [87]. However, ethanol (versus water) washing removes most of the isoflavones and saponins in the process of concentrating the protein.

Background

Soy protein is also consumed as a component of traditional fermented and nonfermented soy foods, such as tofu, tempeh, and miso, as well as whole soybeans, soynuts, soymilk, soy yogurt, and soy cheese. These products contain variable amounts of soy protein and other naturally occurring soy constituents, depending on the specific technologies used in these products. Many soy products, such as tofu, soy nuts, and soy butter, have a high content of PUFAs (see earlier section on PUFAs) and fiber and are low in saturated fat. Soy protein ingredients and soy protein-containing foods may partially replace or be used in addition to animal or other vegetable protein sources in the human diet. Soy protein products are widely available in supermarkets. Persons can achieve an intake of more than 30 g soy protein/day by consuming two or three servings of soy products daily. Examples of the soy content of readily available items include 8 oz soy milk (4–10 g), 4 oz tofu (8–13 g), 1 oz soy flour (10–13 g), 1 oz isolated soy protein (23 g), $\frac{1}{2}$ cup textured soy protein, (11 g), and 3.2 oz meat analogue (18 g).

Studies

Soy and soy isoflavones have been studied extensively, investigating their potential hypocholesterolemic effects and possible role in preventing CAD. The cholesterol-lowering effect of soy protein is attributed to alterations in bile acid and cholesterol absorption, increased LDL receptor activity, or other mechanisms [1]. Several mechanisms have been proposed, including estrogenic effects, modification of LDL receptor activity, or alterations in bile acid or cholesterol absorption. Carroll and Kurowska suggest that the active component in soy may be the protein itself; its benefits presumably result from the amino acid pattern and peptide structure and from nonprotein compounds such as isoflavones and saponins. Cellular and molecular events associated with the formation of fatty streaks and their progression to unstable plaques need further investigation [88].

When substituted for animal protein in the diet, soy protein will lower cholesterol [89–91] in a dose-related matter, most notably in patients with hypercholesterolemia [91]. Anderson et al. demonstrated that a dose-dependent reduction was seen in serum LDL cholesterol concentrations, according to quartiles of the initial serum cholesterol levels, ranging from a clinically nonsignificant 4.4% reduction in subjects with mild hypercholesterolemia (200–255 mg/dl) to a significant 19.6% reduction in subjects with severe hypercholesterolemia (more than 335 mg/dl). Changes in serum TG concentrations were significantly related to the initial serum TG concentrations, but changes in individual quartile groups were not statistically significant. Soy protein did not significantly affect serum HDL or VLDL cholesterol concentrations [90]. In retrospective analysis, these reductions in total and LDL cholesterol may be less attributable to the soy protein and more result from a decrease in saturated fat and cholesterol intake and an increase in polyunsaturated fat intake [91].

Evolution of Recommendations

The body of evidence has transformed recommendations about soy protein consumption over the years. In 1993, the Nutrition Committee of the American Heart Association concluded that the "consumption of vegetable proteins leads to lower cholesterol levels than consumption of animal proteins in rabbits but not in humans [92]." In 1999, however, the U.S. Food and Drug Administration (FDA) approved the health claim that "25 grams of soy protein a day, as part of a diet low in saturated fat and cholesterol, may reduce the risk of heart disease [93]." The FDA also stated that "the evidence did not support a significant role for soy isoflavones in cholesterol-lowering effects of soy protein." In its 2000 Scientific Advisory on soy protein, the American Heart Association concluded that "it is prudent to recommend including soy protein foods in a diet low in saturated fat and cholesterol [91]."

Although earlier research indicated that soy protein, as compared with other proteins, had clinically important favorable effects on LDL cholesterol and other cardiovascular disease (CVD) risk factors, many studies reported during the past 10 years have not confirmed these findings [91,94]. Several studies have demonstrated no difference in fasting lipid levels between otherwise healthy hypercholesterolemic men and women who received soy supplement compared to placebo. [95–98] West et al. studied the effects of soy protein combined with a lipid-lowering diet in men and postmenopausal women, both with and without hormone replacement therapy [97]. In all subgroups, dietary therapy was associated with improved lipid profiles, but soy had no additional effects.

Many clinical trials in humans have examined the effects of soy protein containing intact or depleted isoflavones on lipid profiles; most were small and short term and have inconsistent results [98,99]. The meta-analysis by Zhan et al. of the effects of soy protein-containing isoflavones on the lipid profile, published in 2005, demonstrated an association between intake of soy protein containing isoflavones and changes in lipid concentrations in 70%–90% of trials [99]. Compared to the Anderson et al. 1995 meta-analysis, there was a smaller decrease in total and LDL cholesterol, perhaps because the initial cholesterol levels were lower in this meta-analysis and because the subjects ingested less soy protein. Soy protein containing isoflavones decreased total cholesterol by 3.77%; the pooled estimate of the effects of soy protein intake on LDL-C was a decrease of 5.25%, and on TG was 7.27% [100].

AHA Recommendations: The 2006 AHA Dietary guidelines assert that "consumption of soy protein-rich foods may indirectly reduce CVD risk if they replace animal and dairy products that contain saturated fat and cholesterol [16]." Further, "a very large amount of soy protein, comprising more than half of daily protein intake, may lower LDL cholesterol levels by a few percentage points." However, the summary statement also states that "no

meaningful benefit of soy consumption is evident with regard to HDL cholesterol, triglycerides, or lipoprotein (a) [16]."

Summary: Considering the totality of evidence, daily consumption of soy
products with ≥25 g of soy protein with its associated phytochemicals, fiber,
and polyunsaturated fat intact can improve lipid profiles in hypercholesterolemic individuals. Soy pills and supplements such as isoflavones are not
recommended, as the cholesterol-lowering benefit has only been observed
when the intact soy protein (ISP) is used [101,102]. Soy protein without
the isoflavones appears to be less effective in affecting cholesterol and LDL
levels; consuming isoflavones without soy protein may provide other cardiovascular benefits. The effects of using soy extracts of isoflavones as dietary
supplements are largely unknown and cannot be recommended with the
currently available evidence.

Went Yeast

Went yeast, also known as Chinese red yeast rice, is used to make rice wine, as
a food colorant and preservative, and in traditional Chinese medicine to improve
blood circulation and spleen health and to treat indigestion and diarrhea [101–103].
Red yeast rice is prepared by growing red yeast (*Monascus purpureus*) on rice
to produce a red-colored product [104]. Animal and human studies performed in
China demonstrated that consumption of red yeast rice reduces cholesterol concentrations by 11% to 32% and triacylglycerol concentrations by 12% to 19% [105].
Some strains of Chinese red yeast rice produce compounds called monacolins when
prepared by solid fermentation; monacolin content varies between commercially-
available preparations [103]. Red yeast rice also contains sterols, isoflavones, and
monounsaturated fatty acids [104].

Studies

Heber et al. performed a randomized controlled trial evaluating the cholesterol-
lowering effect of a proprietary Chinese red-yeast-rice supplement known as
Cholestin® (Pharmanex, Simi Valley, CA, USA) [104]. This particular supplement contains nine different monaclins, predominantly monacolin K (also known as
mevinolin and lovastatin), which have the ability to inhibit 3-hydroxy-*e*-
methylglutaryl coenzyme A (HMG-CoA) reductase. A total of 83 subjects (46 men
and 37 women) with baseline cholesterol ranging from 204 to 338 mg/dl completed
the trial. All participants received instruction on the American Heart Association's

Step 1 diet (less than 30% of energy from fat, less than 10% of energy from saturated fat, and less than 300 mg cholesterol/day), and then they were randomly assigned to receive capsules containing 2.4 g red yeast rice daily or rice powder placebo. Total cholesterol, LDL-C, and triacylglycerol concentration decreased significantly (16%, 22%, and 11%, respectively) between baseline, 8 weeks, and 12 weeks in the red-yeast-rice-treated group compared with the placebo-treated group. HDL cholesterol concentrations did not differ significantly within or between groups during the study period. Based on further analysis, the authors also concluded that differences in cholesterol levels were not attributable to differences in dietary intake. There were no significant adverse effects in the study participants.

Cholestin®

Cholestin® is currently sold in the United States as a dietary supplement for healthy adults. It differs from traditional red yeast rice that is sold in Chinese grocery stores in that it is manufactured by growing a single strain of *Monascus purpureus* on rice under carefully controlled conditions that increase the statin content [105]. The package insert instructs users to take a maximum of two capsules twice daily (2.4 g) and warns of possible toxicity related to HMG-CoA inhibitors of the statin class. The monacolin K content in Cholestin® is only 0.2%, or approximately 5 mg, which is comparable to 20–40 mg lovastatin (Mevacor®) [104]. The total amount of statins in 2.4 g Cholestin® is about 10 mg (7–8 mg lovastatin and 2–3 mg of other mevinic acids) [103]. The magnitude of cholesterol lowering observed in the Heber et al. study is significantly greater than expected based on HMG-CoA reductase inhibition alone; thus, other components of Cholestin®, such as flavonoids and sterols, likely contribute to its lipid-lowering effect.

Summary: The findings from clinical trials demonstrating significant and clinically relevant cholesterol reduction using a defined Chinese red yeast rice preparation containing 9 different monacolins cannot be generalized to preparations that do not contain the same levels and profile of monacolins [106]. While the initial data look promising, larger studies of longer duration are needed to better assess the long-term efficacy and safety of went yeast supplementation as a potentially cost-effective lipid-lowering agent. Patients using this product should be monitored for statin-related side effects since this supplement is largely identical to prescription statin drugs.

Garlic

Garlic (*Allium sativum*) has long been purported to reduce serum cholesterol. Epidemiologically, countries whose populations consume higher amounts of garlic tend to have a lower incidence of cardiovascular disease [106]. The cholesterol-lowering ability of garlic has been attributed primarily to alliin [106]. The amount of alliin present in common garlic preparations, including garlic powder tablets, steam-distilled garlic oil capsules, and alcohol-aged garlic liquid, is widely variable. The composition and alliinase activity of garlic powder, which is prepared by dehydrating and pulverizing garlic cloves, is similar to fresh garlic [106]. Aged garlic extract contains antioxidant compounds; in cultured cells, it increases nitric oxide production and decreases inflammatory cytokine production [107]. There is conflicting evidence about the effect of garlic on cardiovascular disease risk factors, including blood pressure, platelet activity, plasma viscosity, and serum lipid levels.

Studies

Multiple studies have evaluated the effects of various garlic supplements on serum lipids, with mixed results. Early trials of garlic preparations mainly supported a lipid-lowering effect [108–110]. Mader conducted a large multicenter study evaluating the lipid-lowering effect of garlic tablets (800 mg/day) versus placebo for 16 weeks. Participants with a higher baseline cholesterol experienced a greater reduction in total cholesterol (14%) compared to participants with lower initial levels of cholesterol (7%) [108]. Notably, early trials that demonstrated a positive effect of garlic on cholesterol levels did not control for factors related to dietary intake [109]. Later, well-designed clinical trials that controlled for dietary intake did not uphold these earlier findings. Simons et al. performed a 30-week, double-blind, random-ized, controlled crossover trail investigating garlic powder (300-mg tablets taken three times a day) versus placebo in 30 hypercholesterolemic individuals who all received 4 weeks of dietary counseling. No significant changes were noted in total cholesterol, LDL-C, or HDL-C with garlic treatment [110].

A meta-analysis of 13 RCTs that included persons with a mean total choles-terol of more than 200 mg/dl demonstrated a modest reduction in total cholesterol levels in subjects who received garlic compared to placebo [111]. Multiple small studies demonstrated that garlic supplements in the form of tablets or powder did not significantly change total cholesterol, LDL-C, HDL-C, or triglycerides compared to placebo [111–116]. Despite conflicting results from studies of garlic supple-ments, garlic is believed to have antiatherosclerotic effects that may be mediated by suppressing LDL oxidation or by other mechanisms [117,118].

Summary: Epidemiologically, garlic consumption appears to be associated with lower rates of cardiovascular disease. However, it is not clear whether this is attributable to garlic as a causative factor in lowering cardiovascular risk, or whether this is an association. Multiple studies evaluating the effects of garlic supplements in the forms of tablets, powder, and oils have had mixed results regarding lipid-lowering effect. Still, garlic is believed to have anti-atherosclerotic effects that may be mediated by other mechanisms. Including garlic as regular part of healthy cooking does not appear to be associated with adverse side effects and may in fact help lower cardiovascular risk through mechanisms not yet understood. Because the results are conflicting, there is no well-established recommendation for the quantity of garlic intake to confer benefit.

Vitamin E

Vitamin E, or alpha-tocopherol, has long been touted as having beneficial effects in the prevention or treatment of cardiovascular disease, dementia, and cancer. Few studies, however, have definitively demonstrated a beneficial role for vitamin E supplementation in reducing serum cholesterol or decreasing more mortality. Conflicting results have been published regarding vitamin E supplementation and risk of cardiovascular events in patients with coronary atherosclerosis.

Studies

A recent review of 19 RCTs that included 135,967 subjects with a mean age of 47 to 84 years compared vitamin E supplementation alone (9 RCTs) or in combination with other vitamins or minerals (10 RCTs) [119,120]. Doses ranged from 16.5 to 2000 IU/day. Overall, vitamin E did not affect all-cause mortality. After adjusting for concomitant use of other vitamins and minerals, high-dose vitamin E (greater than 400 IU/day) was associated with increased mortality, whereas mortality was not increased in the 8 RCTs evaluating low-dose vitamin E (less than 400 IU/day).

The Cambridge Heart Antioxidant Study (CHAOS)

The Cambridge Heart Antioxidant Study (CHAOS) was an earlier randomized controlled trial that involved 2002 patients (84% men; mean age, 62 years) with angiographically confirmed CAD [121]. Patients who had previously taken vitamin supplements containing vitamin E were excluded from the study. Patients were randomly assigned to receive vitamin E 400 IU ($n = 489$) or 800 IU ($n = 546$) or placebo ($n = 967$) and were followed for 510 days. Treatment with vitamin E led to a lower occurrence of nonfatal MI or cardiovascular death compared with placebo [41 events (4%) versus 64 events (7%)]. With an absolute risk reduction (ARR) of 3%, the authors concluded that 38 patients would need to be treated (NNT) with vitamin E for 510 days compared to placebo to prevent one additional major cardiovascular event. There was no difference between the vitamin E and placebo groups for all-cause mortality.

Mechanism

The mechanism by which vitamin E may exert beneficial effects on reducing cardiovascular events is not well understood. One proposed mechanism is through reducing the LDL oxidative susceptibility and decreasing circulating oxidized LDL [122,123]. Multiple studies evaluating the effects of daily vitamin E supplementation have shown no significant alteration in total cholesterol, LDL-C, HDL-C, or triglyceride levels [122,124–127]. Moreover, multiple trials have failed to demonstrate a beneficial effect of antioxidant supplements on cardiovascular disease morbidity and mortality [128].

Summary: At this time, there is insufficient evidence to recommend vitamin E supplementation to lower cholesterol or reduce cardiovascular disease risk. Studies provide little convincing evidence that vitamin E supplementation provides benefit, and there is some evidence that it may be harmful. Conversely, a diet with antioxidant-rich foods is recommended; the mechanism by which dietary antioxidants exert beneficial effects deserves further study.

Coenzyme Q10

Coenzyme Q10 (CoQ10), also known as ubiquinone, is an endogenous antioxidant that functions as an electron carrier in the mitochondrial respiratory chain and plays an important role in the synthesis of adenosine triphosphate [129]. It is packaged into the LDL and VLDL fractions of cholesterol and has been suggested as an important factor in reducing risk for developing atherosclerosis [130]. Lowered blood and tissue concentrations of CoQ10 have been reported in a number of diseases, although it is not clear whether this is the cause or an effect of the disease.

There is concern that HMG Co-A reductase inhibitors may lower CoQ10 levels [130,131]. Mortensen et al. [129] demonstrated that a dose-related significant decline of the total serum level of CoQ10 was found in individuals treated with pravastatin or lovastatin compared to placebo. However, the clinical relevance of studies with similar findings is not clear; some authors postulate that the decrease in CoQ10 levels seen may actually be caused by the overall reduction in LDL-C attributable to statin therapy [132]. Some studies have shown no decrease in plasma CoQ10 levels with statin therapy [129,133,134]. At this time, there is no good evidence to support supplementing statin therapy with CoQ10 [129,135–137].

Summary: Several small studies have demonstrated a small increase in HDL-C with CoQ10 supplementation [135,136]. Other studies have also shown a reduction in lipoprotein a [136] and triglycerides [137,138] with CoQ10 supplementation ranging from 60 mg twice a day [136,137] to 150 mg/day [138]. However, larger trials are required to determine if supplementing the diet with CoQ10 has a definitive role in lowering atherogenic factors and reducing adverse cardiovascular events.

Folic Acid

Hyperhomocystinemia is an independent risk factor for endothelial dysfunction and occlusive vascular disease [138–140]. The Homocysteine Studies Collaboration performed a meta-analysis of prospective observational studies that demonstrated an 11% decreased risk of ischemic heart disease and a 19% decreased risk of stroke associated with a 25% reduction in serum homocysteine concentration [141]. Folic acid reduces plasma homocysteine and may be an important therapy for preventing cardiovascular disease. One hypothesis is that folic acid may improve endothelial function [139,140,142] and reduce arterial stiffness in adults with or without hyperhomocystinemia, which was supported by several small RCTs [140,142]. As discussed further, hyperhomocystinemia may in fact be a marker for vascular disease, rather than a cause of vascular disease. Several large trials convincingly demonstrate that although folic acid supplementation successfully lowers serum homocysteine levels, this reduction is not associated with decreased cardiovascular events.

Studies

Liem et al. studied the role of folic acid supplementation in secondary prevention in patients with known coronary artery disease [142]. They performed an open-label study involving 593 patients with known CAD who were followed for a mean of 24 months. 300 patients received 0.5 mg folic acid/day; 293 were controls; all patients had been on statin therapy for a mean of 3.2 years. The primary endpoint was all-cause mortality and a composite of vascular events. At the end of the study period, patients treated with folic acid had an 18% decrease in plasma homocysteine levels; there was no significant change in the untreated group. The primary endpoint was encountered in 31 (10.3%) patients in the folic acid group and in 28 (9.6%) patients in the control group (RR, 1.05; 95% CI, 0.63–1.75). Thus, despite a significant lowering of homocysteine levels, within 2 years, folic acid does not seem to reduce clinical endpoints in patients with stable CAD who were also on statin treatment. The authors concluded that homocysteine might be a modifiable marker of disease only.

In a subsequent study, Liem et al. evaluated the incidence of recurrent events (death, recurrent MI, stroke, unplanned invasive coronary intervention) in the first year after suffering an MI [143]. Patients with hypercholesterolemia who suffered an MI were randomized to receive fluvastatin alone or with 5 mg folic acid daily. At 1 year, primary endpoints were encountered in 43 patients (31%) given folic acid and 45 patients (31%) in the control group. All separate cardiovascular events were equally distributed between both groups. Total cholesterol levels decreased to a similar extent in the two groups. Folic acid did not demonstrate any beneficial additive effects on cardiovascular mortality or morbidity in post-MI patients with hypercholesterolemia who were treated with statin therapy.

The Heart Outcomes Prevention Evaluation (HOPE) 2 Trial

The Heart Outcomes Prevention Evaluation (HOPE) 2 trial further supported the findings of the aforementioned studies [144]. HOPE-2 was a prevention trial of 5522 patients with vascular disease or diabetes from 13 countries in which 2758 patients were randomly assigned to active treatment with folic acid and vitamins B_6 and B_{12} and 2764 patients were assigned to placebo. The primary study outcome was the composite of death from cardiovascular causes, MI, and stroke. Secondary outcomes included total ischemic events, death from any cause, hospitalization for unstable angina, hospitalization for congestive heart failure, revascularization, cancer incidence, and death from cancer. By the end of the 5-year study, supplementation with folic acid, vitamin B_6, and vitamin B_{12} lowered homocysteine levels significantly. However, there were no significant differences in outcomes between the active treatment and placebo groups: 519 patients (18.8%) in the active treatment group and 547 patients (19.8%) in the placebo group died of cardiovascular causes or had a myocardial infarction or stroke (RR, 0.95; 95% CI, 0.84–1.07; $P = 0.41$). Fewer patients in the active treatment group had a stroke than in the placebo group (4% versus 5.3%; RR, 0.75; 95% CI, 0.59–0.97; $P = 0.03$), but the incidence of fatal stroke was low and not significantly different between both groups. More patients in the active treatment group were hospitalized for unstable angina than in the placebo group, but there were no significant differences between the groups regarding hospitalization for heart failure, revascularization, transient ischemic attack, cancer incidence or deaths from cancer.

The Norwegian Vitamin (NORVIT) Trial

The Norwegian Vitamin (NORVIT) trial evaluated 3749 patients who had suffered an acute myocardial infarction within the previous 7 days to receive one of four treatments: 0.8 mg folic acid, 0.4 mg vitamin B_{12}, and 40 mg vitamin B_6; 0.8 mg folic acid and 0.4 mg vitamin B_{12}; 40 mg vitamin B_6; or placebo [145]. The mean length of follow-up was 36 months. Primary outcomes included new nonfatal and fatal myocardial infarction, nonfatal and fatal stroke, and sudden death attributed to coronary heart disease. Secondary endpoints were myocardial infarction, unstable angina pectoris requiring hospitalization, coronary revascularization, stroke, and death from any cause. The mean homocysteine level was decreased by 27% in the two groups that received folic acid and vitamin B_{12}, but there was no difference in the mean homocysteine level in the group treated with vitamin B_6 alone. Similar to the findings of the HOPE-2 trial, there was no significant beneficial effect on primary or secondary outcomes in individuals with recent myocardial infarction despite lowered serum homocysteine levels through folic acid, vitamin B_6, and vitamin B_{12} supplementation. There was a trend toward increased rate of events in patients receiving folic acid, vitamin B_{12}, and vitamin B_6.

Some studies have demonstrated a beneficial effect of folic acid supplementation on endothelial function [146,147]. However, the clinical significance of these findings is uncertain, particularly in light of the results of studies that have not demonstrated a reduction in cardiovascular events associated with folic acid supplementation.

Summary: At this time, there is no evidence that folic acid supplementation has a role in secondary prevention of clinical cardiovascular events. It may, in fact, be harmful after acute myocardial infarction, and folic acid supplementation is therefore not recommended for the prevention or treatment of cardiovascular disease.

Fenugreek

Fenugreek (*Trigonella foenum-graecum*) is a plant that grows wild from the eastern Mediterranean area to China; it is also cultivated worldwide. It is grown as a potherb (its leaves) and for the spice made from its seeds. The herb contains phytoestrogens, and it has been used in Egypt, India, and the Middle East since ancient times both in cooking and for medicinal purposes. It has long been used as a supplement to increase milk production in lactating women.

Studies

Multiple animal studies and a few small human studies have been conducted evaluating the effect of fenugreek on blood glucose and cholesterol levels. In a 2-month, double-blind study of 25 individuals with newly diagnosed type 2 diabetes, use of 1 g per day of fenugreek extract significantly improved some measures of blood sugar control and insulin response as compared to placebo. Triglyceride levels decreased and HDL cholesterol levels increased, presumably as a consequence of the enhanced insulin sensitivity [148]. The combined results of five randomized controlled trials involving 140 patients that studied the effect of fenugreek seeds on serum cholesterol suggest that total serum cholesterol is reduced between 15% and

33% compared to baseline. Four of these studies were conducted in India, and the methodological quality of four of the studies was considered generally poor [149].

Summary: Larger, methodologically sound studies are needed to ascertain fenugreek's role on serum cholesterol levels. The limited evidence to date suggests that fenugreek may be an effective adjunct in lowering serum cholesterol. The typical dosage is 5 to 30 g of defatted fenugreek taken 3 times a day with meals; 1 gram per day of a water/alcohol fenugreek extract, the dose used in the double-blind study, is another option [150]. Side effects of fenugreek include mild gastrointestinal symptoms such as increased flatulence, nausea, fullness, and diarrhea [149].

Artichoke

Artichoke (*Cynara scolymus*) leaf extract (ALE) is an over-the-counter preparation that is used to lower cholesterol. There are few randomized controlled trials that evaluate the effect of artichoke leaf extract alone (versus as a part of combination treatment) on serum cholesterol. The results of two randomized controlled trials involving 187 patients demonstrated a significant reduction in total cholesterol levels in patients with baseline cholesterol levels greater than 230 mg/dl [150,151]. Another study suggested that dietary supplementation with artichoke extract may improve endothelial function in patients with hypercholesterolemia [152]. ALE appears to be a safe supplement with few reported adverse events: flatulence, hunger, weakness [152].

Summary: Further studies are needed to confirm ALE's hypocholesterolemic role, but it appears to be a safe supplement for lowering cholesterol in patients with moderate hypercholesterolemia.

Myrrh

Herbal extracts from *Commiphora mukul*, also known as myrrh or guggul, have been used in Asia as cholesterol-lowering agents. It is thought that myrrh may exert a lipid-lowering effect by antagonizing two nuclear hormone receptors involved in cholesterol metabolism [153]. Early small studies suggested that myrrh elicits significant reductions in serum total cholesterol (by 10%–27% compared to baseline), low density lipoprotein cholesterol (LDL-C), and triglycerides (TGs), as well as elevations in high-density lipoprotein cholesterol (HDL-C) [149,154].

Studies

A randomized, controlled trial of 103 community-dwelling healthy adults with hypercholesterolemia eating a typical Western diet, in which subjects were randomized to high-dose guggulipid, low-dose guggulipid, or placebo, demonstrated that LDL-C was raised 4% to 5% in the subjects who received guggulipid supplementation. LDL-C was lowered by 5% in the placebo group [154]. Potential side effects include rash, stomach discomfort, rhabdomyolysis, and headache [149,154].

Summary: At this time, there is not enough scientific evidence to support the use of myrrh for hyperlipidemia [154].

Eggplant

The dried powdered fruit of eggplant (*Solanum melongena*) is consumed extensively in Brazil, in a typical dose of 900 mg twice daily, and is believed to have a lipid-lowering effect [155]. However, the results of small clinical trials evaluating the lipid-lowering effect of eggplant powder do not support this belief.

Studies

In one study involving 38 hypercholesterolemic subjects who received either *S. melongena* infusion or placebo for 5 weeks versus dietary counseling alone, there was a modest transitory decrease in total cholesterol and LDL-C in the group who received *S. melongena* infusion. However, after dietary counseling, there were no significant differences between any of the groups regarding any of the parameters [155]. In another randomized, controlled study involving 41 volunteers who were randomized to receive 900 mg dried powdered fruits of eggplant twice daily versus placebo, there was no significant difference in serum lipid levels between groups after 3 months of therapy [156]. A third trial of 21 patients compared the effect of eggplant extract versus lovastatin on serum lipid levels. Baseline lipid levels were similar in each of the study groups: eggplant group, lovastatin group, and control group. After 6 weeks, total cholesterol and LDL-C were lower in the lovastatin group compared to placebo, but there was no statistically significant change in the eggplant group [157].

Summary: At this time, there is not enough scientific evidence to support the use of eggplant for hyperlipidemia.

Holy Basil

Holy basil, also known as sacred basil (*Ocimum tenuiflorum*), is a plant that grows wild in India and is considered sacred by Hindus [158]. It has a long history of medicinal use for such ailments as fever, pain, bronchitis, vomiting, and diseases of the heart and blood, as well as for the treatment of diabetes, arthritis, and asthma. It has also been used for skin diseases and as a prophylactic against malaria.

Holy basil is used in several forms: fresh leaves, leaf juice, and extract [158]. Among its constituents, holy basil contains flavonoids (antioxidants). Holy basil is thought to possess multiple pharmacologic effects, including immunomodulating, hepatoprotective, and antiinflammatory effects. Holy basil has been endowed with myriad attributes: it is touted to improve longevity and promote a healthy life through its rejuvenating, revitalizing, antiseptic, antiallergic, and anticancer effects [158]. As such, holy basil is viewed as an "adaptogen," or an agent that allows the organism to counter adverse physical, chemical, or biological stressors by raising nonspecific resistance toward such stress, thus allowing the organism to "adapt" to the stressful circumstances [158].

Studies assessing holy basil's effect on hyperlipidemia are few. In 1996, Agrawal et al. published a small study evaluating 40 patients with noninsulin-dependent diabetes who received 2.5 g holy basil leaf or placebo powder every morning for 4 weeks; the groups crossed over after 4 weeks [159]. Fasting and postprandial blood glucose and serum cholesterol levels were measured. In addition to a significant reduction in fasting and postprandial glucose (17.6% and 7.3%, respectively), there was a mild reduction in mean total cholesterol during the treatment period. Larger, more recent studies of holy basil on serum lipid levels are lacking.

Summary: At this time, there is not enough scientific evidence to support the use of holy basil for hyperlipidemia. Further studies are needed to shed light on this historically versatile herb.

Author's Summary Recommendations

From the time we are born, food sustains us. Families gather around tables to discuss the day's events, enjoying meals carefully or perhaps hurriedly prepared. An absolutely integral part of our physical health, the food we eat is also a colorful and potentially fun expression of who we are as social beings, underscoring the old adage "we are what we eat."

A diet rich in therapeutic foods should be pleasing to the palate even as it enhances overall health. A truly balanced diet provides an appropriate amount of micro- and macronutrients to complement an active lifestyle and healthy emotional state. "Health" must be viewed not simply as being free from disease, but as a combination of physical, emotional, and spiritual well-being. Primary care physicians are perfectly suited to acknowledge and encourage patients to develop these key components of health.

Putting into perspective the evidence presented in this chapter, this author recommends a diet rich in whole foods—that is, foods that "come in their own package"—such as fruits, nuts, and whole grains. It is unquantifiable just how much health benefit is lost when nature's package is disrupted. When available, whole foods—versus tablets, powders, and oil supplements—should be the primary sources of vitamins, minerals, and antioxidants. Plenty of fruits and vegetables along the "eat the rainbow" mantra to create a "colorful plate" should be the rule, not the exception. A colorful plate contains foods rich in antioxidants and lipid-lowering compounds.

Limit processed foods with simple carbohydrates that stimulate insulin secretion and enhance the appetite. Encourage intake of foods and beverages supplemented with plant sterols and stanols. Replace saturated fat with lean meats, particularly fish rich in omega-3 fatty acids. Cook with monounsaturated oils such as olive oil; polyunsaturated oils such as canola oil are less ideal but acceptable alternatives. Tofu and other sources of soy protein are also good substitutes for saturated fats, providing good sources of protein and antioxidants. Cooking with a variety of herbs and spices, which may have lipid-lowering effects (although further studies are needed to definitively establish this), such as garlic, holy basil, fenugreek, and went yeast, will stimulate the palate without adding unwanted calories. Avoid *trans* fatty acids and saturated fat. Remember to round out the meal with a 5-oz glass of red wine and a small piece of dark chocolate as excellent sources of antioxidant-rich flavonols. These familiar and acquired tastes promise to please the palate. Table 4.1 summarizes the recommendations of the therapeutic foods discussed in this chapter.

References

1. Zarraga IG, Schwarz ER. Impact of dietary patterns and interventions on cardiovascular health. Circulation 2006;114(9):961–973.
2. Marinangeli CP, Varady KA, Jones PJ. Plant sterols combined with exercise for the treatment of hypercholesterolemia: overview of independent and synergistic mechanisms of action. J Nutr Biochem 2006;17(4):217–224.
3. Noakes M, Clifton PM, Doornbos AM, Trautwein EA. Plant sterol ester-enriched milk and yogurt effectively reduce serum cholesterol in modestly hypercholesterolemic subjects. Eur J Nutr 2005;44(4):214–222.
4. Volpe R, Niittynen L, Korpela R, Sirtori C, Bucci A, Fraone N, Pazzucconi F. Effects of yogurt enriched with plant sterols on serum lipids in patients with moderate hypercolesterolemia. Br J Nutr 2001;86(2):233–239.
5. Tikkanen MJ, Hogstrom P, Tuomilehto J, Keinanen-Kiukaanniemi S, Sundvall J, Karppanen H. Effect of a diet based on a low-fat foods enriched with nonesterified plant sterols and mineral nutrients on serum cholesterol. Am J Cardiol 2001;88(10):1157–1162.
6. Pouteau EB, Monnard IE, Piguet-Welsch C, Groux MJ, Sagalowicz L, Berger A. Non-esterified plant sterols solubilized in low fat milks inhibit cholesterol absorption—a stable isotope double-blind crossover study. Eur J Nutrition 2003;42(3):154–164.

7. Thomsen AB, Hansen HB, Christiansen C, Green H, Berger A. Effect of free plant sterols in low-fat milk on serum lipid profile in hypercholesterolemic subjects. Eur J Clin Nutr 2004;58(6):860–870.

8. Devaraj S, Jialal I, Vega-Lopez S. Plant sterol-fortified orange juice effectively lowers cholesterol levels in mildly hypercholesterolemic healthy individuals. Arterioscler Thromb Vasc Biol 2004;24(3):e-25–e-28.

9. Hendriks HFJ, Westrate JA, van Vliet T, Meijer GW. Spreads enriched with three different levels of vegetable oil sterols and the degree of cholesterol lowering in normocholesterolaemic and mildly hypercholesterolaemic subjects. Eur J Clin Nutr 1999;53:319–327.

10. Jones PJ, Ntanios FY, Raeini-Sarjaz M, Vanstone CA. Cholesterol-lowering efficacy of a sitostanol-containing phytosterol mixture with a prudent diet in hyperlipidemic men. Am J Clin Nutr 1999;69:1144–1150.

11. Miettinen TA, Puska P, Gylling H, Vanhanen H, Vartianinen E. Reduction of serum cholesterol with sitostanol-ester margarine in a mildly hypercholesterolemic population. N Engl J Med 1995;333:1308–1312.

12. Jones PJ, Raeini-Sarjaz M, Ntanios FY, Vanstone CA, Feng JY, Parsons WE. Modulation of plasma lipid levels and cholesterol kinetics by phytosterol versus phytostanol esters. J Lipid Res 2000;41:697–705.

13. Gylling H, Miettinen TA. Cholesterol reduction by different plant stanol mixtures and with variable fat intake. Metabolism 1999;48:575–580.

14. Lichtenstein AH, Appel LJ, Brands M, et al. Diet and lifestyle recommendations revision 2006: a scientific statement from the American Heart Association nutrition committee. Circulation 2006;113:82–96.

15. Amundsen AL, Ntanios F, Put N, Ose L. Long-term compliance and changes in plasma lipids, plant sterols and carotenoids in children and parents with FH consuming plant sterol ester-enriched spread. Eur J Clin Nutr 2004;58(12):1612–1620.

16. Sierksma A, Weststrate JA, Meijer GW. Spreads enriched with plant sterols, either esterified 4,4-dimethylsterols or free 4-desmethylsterols, and plasma total- and LDL-cholesterol concentrations. Br J Nutr 1999;82:273–282.

17. Christiansen LI, Lahteenmake PL, Mannelin MR, Seppanen-Laakso TE, Hiltunen RV, Yliruusi K. Cholesterol-lowering effect of spreads enriched with microcrystalline plant sterols in hypercholesterolemic subjects. Eur J Clin Nutr 2001;40(2):66–73.

18. Korpela R, Tuomilehto J, Hogstrom P, et al. Safety aspects and cholesterol-lowering efficacy of low fat dairy products containing plant sterols. Eur J Clin Nutr 2006;60(5):633–642.

19. Vau VW, Journoud M, Jones PJ. Plant sterols are efficacious in lowering plasma LDL and non-HDL cholesterol in hypercholesterolemic type 2 diabetic and nondiabetic persons. Am J Clin Nutr 2005;81(6):1351–1358.

20. de Jongh S, Vissers MN, Rol P, et al. Plant sterols lower LDL cholesterol without improving endothelial function in prepubertal children with familial hypercholesterolemia. J Inherit Metab Dis 2003;26(4):343–351.

21. Amundsen AL, Ntanios F, Put N, et al. Long-term compliance and changes in plasma lipids, plant sterols and carotenoids in children and parents with FH consuming plant sterol ester-enriched spread. Eur J Clin Nutr 2004;58(12):1612–1620.

22. Moruisi KG, Oosthuizen W, Opperman AM. Phytosterols/stanols lower cholesterol concentrations in familial hypercholesterolemic subjects: a systematic review with meta-analysis. J Am Coll Nutr 2006;25(1):41–48.

23. O'Neill FH, Brynes A, Mandeno R, et al. Comparison of the effects of dietary plant sterol and stanol esters on lipid metabolism. Nutr Metab Cardiovasc Dis 2004;14(3):133–142.

24. Miettinen TA, Gylling H. Plant stanol and sterol esters in prevention of cardiovascular diseases. Ann Med 2004;36(2):126–134.

25. Goldberg AC, Ostlund RE, Bateman JH, et al. Effect of plant stanol tablets on low-density lipoprotein cholesterol lowering in patients on statin drugs. Am J Cardiol 2006;97(3): 376–379.

26. Thompson GR. Additive effects of plant sterol and stanol esters to statin therapy. Am J Cardiol 2005;96(1A):37D–39D.

27. Cater NM, Garcia-Garcia AB, Vega GL, et al. Responsiveness of plasma lipids and lipoproteins to plant stanol esters. Am J Cardiol 2005;96(1A):23D–28D.

28. Katan MB, Grundy SM, Jones P, et al. Efficacy and safety of plant stanols and sterols in the management of blood cholesterol levels. Mayo Clinic Proc 2003;78(8):965–978.

29. Jakulj L, Trip MD, Sudhop T, et al. Inhibition of cholesterol absorption by the combination of dietary plant sterols and ezetimibe: effects on plasma lipid levels. J Lipid Res 2005;46(12):2692–2698.

30. Grundy SM. Stanol esters as a component of maximal dietary therapy in the National Cholesterol Education Program Adult Treatment Panel III Report. Am J Cardiol 2005;96(1A): 47D–50D.

31. Patch CS, Tapsell LC, Williams PG. Plant sterol/stanol prescription is an effective treatment strategy for managing hypercholesterolemia in outpatient clinical practice. J Am Diet Assoc 2005;105(1):46–52.

32. Gruppo Italiano per lo Studio della Sopravvivenza nell'Infarto miocardico (GISSI)-Prevenzione Investigators. Dietary supplementation with n-3 polyunsaturated fatty acids and vitamin E after myocardial infarction: results of the GISSI-Prevenzione Trial. Lancet 1999; 354: 447–455.

33. Marchioli R, Barzi F, Bomba E, et al., on behalf of the GISSI-Prevenzione Investigators. Early protection against sudden death by n-3 fatty acids after myocardial infarction: time course analysis of the results of the Gruppo Italiano per lo Studio della Sopravvivenza nell'Infarto miocardico (GISSI)-Prevenzione. Circulation 2002;105:1897–1903.

34. Macchia A, Levantesi G, Franzosi MG, et al. Left ventricular systolic dysfunction, total mortality, and sudden death in patients with myocardial infarction treated with n-3 polyunsaturated fatty acids. Eur J Heart Fail 2005;7:904–909.

35. Singh RB, Niaz MA, Sharma JP, et al. Randomized, double-blind, placebo-controlled trial of fish oil and mustard oil in patients with suspected acute myocardial infarction: the Indian experiment of infarct survival. Cardiovasc Drugs Ther 1997;11:485–491.

36. Yokoyama M, Origasa H, for the JELIS Investigators. Effects of eicosapentaenoic acid on cardiovascular events in Japanese patients with hypercholesterolemia: rationale, design, and baseline characteristics of the Japan EPA Lipid Intervention Study (JELIS). Am Heart J 2003;146:613–620.

37. Jacobson TA. Secondary prevention of coronary artery disease with omega-3 fatty acids. Am J Cardiol 2006;98(suppl):61i–70i. Accessed from www.AJConline.org 6 Sep 06.

38. Burr ML, Fehily AM, Gilbert JF, et al. Effects of changes in fat, fish, and fiber intake on death and myocardial infarction: Diet and Reinfarction Trial (DART). Lancet 1989;334: 757–761.

39. Albert CM, Gaziano MJ, Willet WC, et al. Nut consumption and decreased risk of sudden cardiac death in the Physicians' Health Study. Arch Intern Med 2002;162:1382–1387.

40. Studer M, Brief M, Leimenstoll B, et al. Effect of different antilipidemic agents and diets on mortality: a systematic review. Arch Intern Med 2005;165:725–730.

41. Bucher HC, Hengstler P, Schindler C, et al. n-3 polyunsaturated fatty acids in coronary heart disease: a meta-analysis of randomized controlled trials. Am J Med 2002;112:298–304.

42. Nilsen DW, Albrektsen G, Landmark K, et al. Effects of a high-dose concentrate of n-3 fatty acids or corn oil introduced early after an acute myocardial infarction on serum triacylglycerol and HDL cholesterol. Am J Clin Nutr 2001;74:50–56.

43. Siscovick DS, Raghunathan T, King I, et al. Dietary intake of long-chain omega-3 polyunsaturated fatty acids and risk of primary cardiac arrest. Am J Clin Nutr 2000;71(suppl): 208S–212S.

44. Leaf A, Xiao YF, Kang JX, et al. Prevention of sudden cardiac death by omega-3 polyunsaturated fatty acids. Pharmacol Ther 2003;98:355–377.

45. Hooper L, Thompson RL, Harrison RA, et al. Risks and benefits of omega 3 fats for mortality, cardiovascular disease, and cancer: systematic review. BMJ 2006;332:752–760.

46. Calo L, Bianconi L, Colivicchi F, et al. n-3 fatty acids for the prevention of atrial fibrillation after coronary artery bypass surgery: a randomized, controlled trial. J Am Coll Cardiol 2005;45:1723–1728.

47. Brouwer IA, Zock PL, Wever EF, et al. Rationale and design of a randomized controlled clinical trial on supplemental intake of omega-3 fatty acids and incidence of cardiac arrhythmia: SOFA. Eur J Clin Nutr 2003;57:1323–1330.

48. Leaf A, Albert CM, Josephson M, et al., for the Fatty Acid Antiarrhythmia Trial Investigators. Prevention of fatal arrhythmias in high-risk subjects by fish oil n-3 fatty acid intake. Circulation 2005;112:2762–2768.

49. Raitt MH, Connor WE, Morris C, et al. Fish oil supplementation and risk of ventricular tachycardia and ventricular fibrillation in patients with implantable defibrillators: a randomized controlled trial. JAMA 2005;293:2884–2891.

50. Leaf A, Kang JX, Xiao YF, et al. n-3 fatty acids in the prevention of cardiac arrhythmias. Lipids 1999;34(suppl):S187–S189.

51. Expert Panel on Detection, Evaluation, and Treatment of High Blood Cholesterol in Adults. Executive Summary of the Third Report of the National Cholesterol Education Program (NCEP) Expert Panel Detection, Evaluation, and Treatment of High Blood Cholesterol in Adults. JAMA 2001; 285:2486–2497.

52. US Food and Drug Administration, Center for Food Safety and Applied Nutrition. Letter regarding dietary supplement health claim for omega-3 fatty acids and coronary heart disease. October 31, 2000. [http://www.cfsan.fda.gov/~dms/dr-ltr11.html.]

53. Kris-Etherton PM, Harris WS, Appel LJ, for the Nutrition Committee. Fish consumption, fish oil, omega-3 fatty acids, and cardiovascular disease. Circulation 2002;106:2747–2757.

54. Scandale S, Lee DT, Harris WS. Omega-3 fatty acids: fish oil use in primary care practice. Fam Pract Recert 2006;28:20–31.

55. Harris WS. Fish oil supplementation: evidence for health benefits. Clevel Clin J Med 2004;71:208–221.

56. www.omacorrx.com, accessed 6 October 2006.

57. Kris-Etherton PM, Derr JA, Mustad VA, Seligson FH, Pearson TA. Effects of a milk chocolate bar per day substituted for a high-carbohydrate snack in young men on an NCEP/AHA Step 1 Diet. Am J Clin Nutr 1994;60(6 suppl):1037S–1042S.

58. Wan Y, Vinson JA, Etherton TD, et al. Effects of coca powder and dark chocolate on LDL oxidative susceptibility and prostaglandin concentrations in humans. Am J Clin Nutr 2001;74(5):596–602.

59. De Graaf J, De Sauvage Nolting PR, Van Dam M, et al. Consumption of tall oil-derived phytosterols in a chocolate matrix significantly decreases plasma total and low-density lipoprotein-cholesterol levels. Br J Nutr 2002;88(5):479–488.

60. Mursu J, Voutilainen S, Nurmi T, et al. Dark chocolate consumption increases HDL cholesterol concentration and chocolate fatty acids may inhibit lipid peroxidation in healthy humans. Free Radic Biol Med 2004;37(9):1351–1359.

61. Ding EL, Hutfless SM, Ding X, et al. Chocolate and prevention of cardiovascular disease: a systematic review. Nutr Metab 2006;3:1–12. Accessed from http://www.nutritionandmetabolism.com/content/3/1/2 on 16 Sep 06.

62. Hirano R, Osakabe N, Iwamoto A, et al. Antioxidant effects of polyphenols in chocolate on low-density lipoprotein both in vitro and ex vivo. J Nutr Sci Vitaminol 2000;46(4):199–204.

63. Mensink RP, Zock PL, Kester AD, et al. Effects of dietary fatty acids and carbohydrates on the ratio of serum total to HDL cholesterol and on serum lipids and apolipoproteins: a meta-analysis of 60 controlled trials. Am J Clin Nutr 2003;77:1146–1155.

64. Franco OH, Bonneux L, de Laet C, et al. The Polymeal: a more natural, safer, and probably tastier (than the Polypill) strategy to reduce cardiovascular disease by more than 75 percent. BMJ 2004;329:1447–1450.

65. Jenkins DJ, Kendall CW, Vuksan V, et al. Soluble fiber intake at a dose approved by the US Food and Drug Administration for a claim of health benefits: serum lipid risk factors for cardiovascular disease assessed in a randomized controlled crossover trial. Am J Clin Nutr 2002;75(5):834–839.

66. Brown L, Rosner B, Willett WW, et al. Cholesterol-lowering effects of dietary fiber: a meta-analysis. Am J Clin Nutr 1999;69(1):30–42.

67. Anderson JW, Allgood LD, Lawrence A, et al. Cholesterol-lowering effects of psyllium intake adjunctive to diet therapy in men and women with hypercholesterolemia: a meta-analysis of 8 controlled trials. Am J Clin Nutr 2000;71(2):472–479.

68. Aller R, de Luis DA, Izaola O, et al. Effect of soluble fiber intake in lipid and glucose levels in healthy subjects: a randomized clinical trial. Diabetes Res Clin Pract 2004;65(1):7–11.

69. Olson BH, Anderson SM, Becker MP, et al. Psyllium-enriched cereals lower blood total cholesterol and LDL cholesterol, but not HDL cholesterol, in hypercholesterolemic adults: results of a meta-analysis. J Nutr 1997;127(10):1973–1980.

70. Bell LP, Hectorn KJ, Reynolds H, et al. Cholesterol-lowering effects of soluble fiber cereals as part of a prudent diet for patients with mild to moderate hypercholesterolemia. Am J Clin Nutr 1990;52(6):1020–1026.

71. Williams CL, Bollella M, Spark A, et al. Soluble fiber enhances the hypocholesterolemic effect of the step I diet in childhood. J Am Coll Nutr 1995;14(3):251–257.

72. Behall KM, Scholfield DJ, Hallfrisch J. Lipids significantly reduced by diets containing barley in moderately hypercholesterolemic men. J Am Coll Nutr 2004;23(1):55–62.

73. Behall KM, Scholfield DJ, Hallfrisch J. Diets containing barley significantly reduce lipids in mildly hypercholesterolemic men and women. Am J Nutr 2004;80(5):1185–1193.

74. Moreyra AE, Wilson AC, Koraym A. Effect of combining psyllium fiber with simvastatin in lowering cholesterol. Arch Intern Med 2005;165(10):1161–1166.

75. Karmally W, Montez MG, Palmas W, et al. Cholesterol-lowering benefits of oat-containing cereal in Hispanic Americans. J Am Diet Assoc 2005;105(6):967–970.

76. Chen J, He J, Wildman RP, et al. A randomized controlled trial of dietary fiber intake on serum lipids. Eur J Clin Nutr 2006;60(1):62–68.

77. Carmago CA, Stampher MJ, Glynn RJ, et al. Moderate alcohol consumption and risk for angina pectoris and myocardial infarction in male US physicians. Ann Intern Med 1997;126:372–375.

78. Renaud SC, Guegen R, Siest G, et al. Wine, beer, and mortality in middle-aged men for Eastern France. Arch Intern Med 1999;159:1865–1870.

79. Klatsky AL, Armstrong MA, Friedman GD. Alcohol and mortality. Ann Intern Med 1992;117:646–654.

80. Gronbaek M, Becker U, Johansen D, et al. Type of alcohol consumed and mortality from all causes, coronary disease and cancer. Ann Intern Med 2000;133:411–419.

81. Di Catelnuovo A, Rotondo S, Iacoviello L, et al. Meta-analysis of wine and beer consumption in relation to vascular risk. Circulation 2002;105:2836–2844.

82. St Leger AS, Cochrane AL, Moore F. Factors associated with cardiac mortality in developed countries with particular reference to consumption of wine. Lancet 1979;12:1017–1020.

83. Groenback M, Deis A, Sorensen T, et al. Mortality associated with moderate intakes of wine, beer or spirits. BMJ 1995;310:1165.

84. Goldfinger TM. Beyond the French Paradox: the impact of moderate alcohol and wine consumption in the prevention of cardiovascular disease. Cardiol Clin 2003;21:449–457.

85. Maxwell S, Cruickshank A, Thorpe G. Red wine and antioxidant activity in serum. Lancet 1994;344:193–194.

86. Erdman JW. Soy protein and cardiovascular disease: a statement for healthcare professionals from the nutrition committee of the AHA. Circulation 2000;102;2555–2559.

87. Protein Technologies International. Soy protein and health: discovering a role for soy protein in the fight against coronary heart disease. Houston, TX: Marimac Communications, 1996.

88. Carroll KK, Kurowska EM. Soy consumption and cholesterol reduction: review of animal and human studies. J Nutr 1995;125(suppl):594S–597S.

89. Potter SM. Soy protein and cardiovascular disease: the impact of bioactive components in soy. Nutr Rev 1998;56(8):231–235.

90. Anderson JW, Johnstone BM, Cook-Newell ME. Meta-analysis of the effects of soy protein intake on serum lipids. N Engl J Med 1995;333:276–282.

91. Sacks FM, Lichtenstein A, Van Horn L, et al. Soy protein, isoflavones, and cardiovascular health: an American Heart Association science advisory for professionals from the Nutrition Committee. Circulation 2006;113:1034–1044.

92. Chait A, Brunzell JD, Denke MA, et al. Rationale of the diet–heart statement of the American Heart Association: report of the Nutrition Committee. Circulation 1993;88: 3008–3029.

93. Food and Drug Administration. Food labeling: health claims: soy protein and coronary heart disease. 21 CFR Part 101. Fed Reg 1999; 64:57700–57733.

94. Dewell A, Hollenbeck PL, Hollenbeck CB. Clinical review: a critical evaluation of the role of soy protein and isoflavone supplementation in the control of plasma cholesterol concentrations. J Clin Endocrinol Metab 2006;91(3):772–780.

95. Ma Y, Chiriboga D, Olendzki BC, et al. Effect of soy protein containing isoflavones on blood lipids in moderately hypercholesterolemic adults: a randomized controlled trial. J Am Coll Nutr 2005;24(4):275–285.

96. Hermansen K, Hansen B, Jacobsen R, et al. Effects of soy supplementation on blood lipids and arterial function in hypercholesterolemic subjects. Eur J Clin Nutr 2005;59(7):843–850.

97. West SG, Hilpert KF, Juturu V, et al. Effects of including soy protein in a blood cholesterol-lowering diet on markers of cardiac risk in men and in postmenopausal women with and without hormone replacement therapy. J Women's Health 2005;14(3):253–262.

98. Cuevas AM, Irribarra VL, Castillo OA, Yanez MD, Germain AM. Isolated soy protein improves endothelial function in postmenopausal hypercholesterolemic women. Eur J Clin Nutr 2003;57(8):889–894.

99. Zhan S, Ho SC. Meta-analysis of the effects of soy protein containing isoflavones on the lipid profile. Am J Clin Nutr 2005;81:397–408.

100. Zhuo XG, Melby MK, Watanabe S. Soy isoflavone intake lowers serum LDL cholesterol: a meta-analysis of 8 randomized controlled trials in humans. J Nutr 2004;134(9):2395–2400.

101. Dunn AV. Incorporating soy protein into a low-fat, low-cholesterol diet. Clevel Clin J Med 2000;67(10):767–772.

102. Caron MF, White CM. Evaluation of the antihyperlipidemic properties of dietary supplements. Pharmacotherapy 2001;21(4):481–487.

103. Havel RJ. Dietary supplement or drug? The case of Cholestin. Am J Clin Nutr 1999;69: 175–176.

104. Heber D, Yip I, Ashley JM, et al. Cholesterol-lowering effects of a proprietary Chinese red-yeast-rice dietary supplement. Am J Clin Nutr 1999;69:231–236.

105. Heber D, Lembertas A, Lu Q, et al. An analysis of nine proprietary Chinese red yeast rice dietary supplements: implications of variability in chemical profile and contents. J Altern Complement Med 2001;7(2):133-139.

106. Spigelski D, Jones PH. Efficacy of garlic supplementation in lowering serum cholesterol levels. Nutr Rev 2001;59:236–244.

107. Williams MJ, Sutherland WH, McCormick MP, Yeoman DJ, deJong SA. Aged garlic extract improves endothelial function in men with coronary artery disease. Phytother Res 2005;19(4):314–319.

108. Mader FH. Treatment of hyperlipidaemia with garlic-powder tablets. Evidence from the German Association of General Practitioners' multicentric placebo-controlled double-blind study. Arzneim-Forsch 1990;40(10):1111–1116.

109. De ASOS, Grunwald J. Effect of garlic powder tablets on blood lipids and blood pressure—a six month placebo controlled, double-blind study. Br J Clin Res 1993;4:37–44.

110. Simons LA, Balasubramaniam S, von Konigsmark M, Parfitt A, Simons J, Peters W. On the effect of garlic on plasma lipids and lipoproteins in mild hypercholesterolemia. Atherosclerosis 1995;113(2):219–225.

111. Stevinson C, Pittler MH, Ernst E. Garlic for treating hypercholesterolemia. A meta-analysis of randomized clinical trials. Ann Intern Med 2000;133(6):420–429.

112. Superko HR, Krauss RM. Garlic powder, effect on plasma lipids, postprandial lipemia, low-density lipoprotein particle size, high-density lipoprotein subclass distribution and lipoprotein (a). J Am Coll Cardiol 2000;35(2):321–326.

113. Isaacsohn JL, Moser M, Stein EA, et al. Garlic powder and plasma lipids and lipoproteins: a multicenter, randomized, placebo-controlled trial. Arch Intern Med 1998;158(11): 1189–1194.

114. Berthold HK, Sudhop T, von Bergmann K. Effect of a garlic oil preparation on serum lipoproteins and cholesterol metabolism: a randomized controlled trial. JAMA 1998;279(23):1900–1902.

115. Peleg A, Hershcovici T, Lipa R, et al. Effect of garlic on lipid profile and psychopathologic parameters in people with mild to moderate hypercholesterolemia. Isr Med Assoc J 2003;5(9):637–640.

116. Jain AK, Vargas R, Gotzkowsky S, et al. Can garlic reduce levels of serum lipids? A controlled clinical study. Am J Med 1993;94(6):632–635.

117. Turner B, Molgaard C, Marckmann P. Effect of garlic (*Allium sativum*) powder tablets on serum lipids, blood pressure, and arterial stiffness in normolipidemic volunteers; a randomized, double-blind, placebo-controlled trial. Br J Nutr 2004;92(4):701–706.

118. Lau BH. Suppression of LDL oxidation by garlic. J Nutr 2001;131(3s):985S–988S.

119. Review: High-dose vitamin E supplementation is associated with increased all-cause mortality. ACP J Club 2005;143(1):1.

120. Vitamin E reduced the risk of cardiovascular events in coronary atherosclerosis. ACP J Club 1996;125:15.

121. Hodis HN, Mack WJ, LaBree L, et al. Alpha-tocopherol supplementation in healthy individuals reduces low-density lipoprotein oxidation but not atherosclerosis: the Vitamin E Atherosclerosis Prevention Study (VEAPS). Circulation 2002;106(12):1453–1459.

122. de Waart FG, Moser U, Kok FJ. Vitamin E supplementation in elderly lowers the oxidation rate of linoleic acid in LDL. Atherosclerosis 1997;133(2):255–263.

123. Stampfer MJ, Willett W, Castelli WP, Taylor JO, Fine J, Hennekens CH. Effect of vitamin E on lipids. Am J Clin Pathol 1983;79(6):714–716.

124. Meydani SN, Meydani M, Rall LC, Morrow F, Blumberg JB. Assessment of the safety of high-dose, short-term supplementation with vitamin E in healthy older adults. Am J Clin Nutr 1994;60(5):704–709.

125. Mensink RP, van Houwelingen AC, Kromhout D, Hornstra G. A vitamin E concentrate rich in tocotrienols had no effect on serum lipids, lipoproteins, or platelet function in men with mildly elevated serum lipid concentrations. Am J Clin Nutr 1999;69(2): 21321–21329.

126. Michcletta F, Natoli S, Misuraca M, et al. Vitamin E supplementation in patients with carotid atherosclerosis: reversal of altered oxidative stress status in plasma but not in plaque. Arterioscler Thromb Vasc Biol 2004;24(1):136–140.

127. Kris-Etherton PM, Lichtenstein AH, Howard BV, et al. AHA Scientific Advisory: antioxidant vitamin supplements and cardiovascular disease. Circulation 2004;110:637–641.

128. Bleske BE, Willis RA, Anthony M, Casselberry N, Datwani M, Uhley VE, Secontine SG, Shea MJ. The effect of pravastatin and atorvastatin on coenzyme Q10. Am Heart J 2001;142(2):E2.

129. Mortensen SA, Leth A, Agner E, et al. Dose-related decrease of serum coenzyme Q10 during treatment with HMG-CoA reductase inhibitors. Mol Aspects Med 1997;18(suppl): S137–S144.

130. Strey CH, Young JM, Molyneux SL, George PM, Florkowski CM, Scott RS, Framton CM. Endothelium-ameliorating effects of statin therapy and coenzyme Q10 reductions in chronic heart failure. Atherosclerosis 2005;179(1):201–206.
131. Human JA, Ubbink JB, Jerling JJ, et al. The effect of simvastatin on the plasma antioxidant concentrations in patients with hypercholesterolemia. Clin Chim Acta 1997;263(1):67–77.
132. Hargreaves IP. Ubiquinone: cholesterol's reclusive cousin. Ann Clin Biochem 2003;40:207–218.
133. Laaksonen R, Jokelainen K, Laakso J, et al. The effect of simvastatin treatment on natural antioxidants in low-density lipoproteins and high-energy phosphates and ubiquinone in skeletal muscle. Am J Cardiol 1996;77(1):851–854.
134. Palomaki A, Malminiemi K, Solakivi T, et al. Ubiquinone supplementation during lovastatin treatment: effect on LDL oxidation ex vivo. J Lipid Res 1998;39(7):1430–1437.
135. Singh RB, Niaz MA. Serum concentration of lipoprotein(a) decreased on treatment with hydrosoluble coenzyme Q10 in patients with coronary artery disease: discovery of a new role. Int J Cardiol 1999;68(1):23–29.
136. Singh RB, Niaz MA, Rastogi SS, et al. Effect of hydrosoluble coenzyme Q10 on blood pressures and insulin resistance in hypertensive patients with coronary artery disease. J Hum Hypertens 1999;13(3):203–208.
137. Cicero AF, Deorsa G, Miconi A, et al. Treatment of massive hypertriglyceridemia resistant to PFUA and fibrates: a possible role for the coenzyme Q10? Biofactors 2005;23(1):7–14.
138. Woo KS, Chook P, Lolin YI, et al. Folic acid improves arterial endothelial function in adults with hyperhomocystinemia. J Am Coll Cardiol 1999;34(7):2002–2006.
139. Liem A, Reynierse-Buitenwerf GH, Zwinderman AH, et al. Secondary prevention with folic acid: effects on clinical outcomes. J Am Coll Cardiol 2003;41(12):2105–2113.
140. Williams C, Kingwell BA, Burke K, et al. Folic acid supplementation for 3 weeks reduces pulse pressure and large artery stiffness independent of MTHFR (methylenentetrahydrofolate reductase) genotype. Am J Clin Nutr 2005;82(1):26–31.
141. Homocysteine Studies Collaboration. Homocysteine and risk of ischemic heart disease and stroke: a meta-analysis. JAMA 2002;288:2015–2022.
142. Liem AH, van Boven AJ, Veeger NJ, et al. Efficacy of folic acid when added to statin therapy in patients with hypercholesterolemia following acute myocardial infarction: a randomized pilot trial. Int J Cardiol 2004;93(2-3):175–179.
143. Lekakis JP, Papamichael CM, Papaioannou TG, et al. Oral folic acid enhances endothelial function in patients with hypercholesterolemia receiving statins. Eur J Cardiovasc Prev Rehabil 2004;11(5):416–420.
144. The Heart Outcomes Prevention Evaluation (HOPE) 2 Investigators. Homocysteine lowering with folic acid and B vitamins in vascular disease. N Engl J Med 2006;354:1567–1577.
145. Bønaa KH, Njølstad I, Ueland PM, et al. Homocysteine lowering and cardiovascular events after acute myocardial infarction. N Engl J Med 2006;354:1778–1788.
146. Verhaar MC, Wever RM, Kastelein JJ, et al. Effects of oral folic acid supplementation on endothelial function in familial hypercholesterolemia. A randomized placebo-controlled trial. Circulation 1999;100(4):335–338.
147. Gupta A, Gupta R, Lal B. Effect of Trigonella foenum-graecum (fenugreek) seeds on glycemic control and insulin resistance in type 2 diabetes mellitus: a double blind placebo controlled study. J Assoc Phys India 2001;49:1057–1061.
148. Thompson C, Joanna S, Ernst E. Herbs for serum cholesterol reduction: a systematic review. J Fam Pract 2003;52(6):468–478.
149. http://healthresources.caremark.com/GetHerbContent.do?primerid=100226929&name=Fenugreek, accessed 16 Sep 06.
150. Pittler MH, Thompson Coon J, Ernst E. Artichoke leaf extract for treating hypercholesterolemia. Cochrane Database Syst Rev 2006;2.
151. Englisch W, Beckers C, Unkauf M, et al. Efficacy of artichoke dry extract in patients with hyperlipoproteinemia. Arzneim-Forsch 2000;50(3):260–265.

152. Lupattelli G, Marchesi S, Lombardini R, Roscini AR, Trinca F, Gemelli F, Vaudo G, Mannarino E. Artichoke juice improves endothelial function in hyperlipemia. Life Sci 2004;76(7):775–782.

153. Szapary PO, Wolfe ML, Bloedon LT, et al. Guggulipid for the treatment of hypercholesterolemia: a randomized controlled trial. JAMA 2003;290(6):765–772.

154. Ulbrict C, Basch E, Szapary P, et al. Guggul for hyperlipidemia: a review by the Natural Standard Research Collaboration. Complement Ther Med 2005;13(4):279–290.

155. Guimarae PR, Galvao AM, Batista CM, et al. Eggplant (*Solanum melongena*) infusion has a modest and transitory effect on hypercholesterolemic subjects. Braz J Med Biol Res 2000;33(9):1027–1036.

156. Silva GE, Takahashi MH, Eik Filho W, et al. Absence of hypolipidemic effect of *Solanum melongena* (eggplant) on hyperlipidemic patients. Arq Bras Endocrinol Metabol 2004;48(3):368–373.

157. Praca JM, Thomaz A, Caramelli B. Eggplant (*Solanum melongena*) extract does not alter serum lipid levels. Arq Bras Cardiol 2004;82(3):269–276.

158. Botanical Pathways. Downloaded on 16 Nov 06.

159. Agrawal P, Rai V, Singh RB. Randomized placebo-controlled, single blind trial of holy basil leaves in patients with noninsulin-dependent diabetes mellitus. Int J Clin Pharmacol Ther 1996;34:406–409.

Suggested Key Readings

Bucher HC, Hengstler P, Schindler C, et al. n-3 polyunsaturated fatty acids in coronary heart disease: a meta-analysis of randomized controlled trials. Am J Med 2002;112: 298–304.

Di Catelnuovo A, Rotondo S, Iacoviello L, et al. Meta-analysis of wine and beer consumption in relation to vascular risk. Circulation 2002;105: 2836–2844.

Ding EL, Hutfless SM, Ding X, et al. Chocolate and prevention of cardiovascular disease: a systematic review. Nutr Metab 2006;3: 1–12. Accessed from: http://www.nutritionandmetabolism.com/content/3/1/2 on 16 Sep 06.

Sacks FM, Lichtenstein A, VanHorn L, et al. Soy protein, isoflavones, and cardiovascular health: an American Heart Association science advisory for professionals from the Nutrition Committee. Circulation 2006;113: 1034–1044.

Thompson C, Joanna S, Ernst E. Herbs for serum cholesterol reduction: a systematic review. J Fam Pract 2003;52(6): 468–478.

Chapter 5
Exercise Interventions to Reduce Lipids and Cardiovascular Disease Risk

Allyson S. Howe and Christopher G. Jarvis

Introduction

Cardiovascular disease (CVD) is the leading cause of death in the United States [1]. The lifetime risk of CVD was evaluated by the Framingham Heart Study and found to be 40% to 49% in men and 32% in women aged 40 to 94 years old [2]. Prospective data demonstrate conclusively that exercise reduces the incidence of coronary artery disease [3,4].

Elevated serum cholesterol and an increased risk of atherosclerotic cardiovascular disease (ASCVD) have been clearly linked [5,6]. Strategies to improve serum cholesterol patterns focus on lifestyle changes in diet and exercise as well as cholesterol-lowering medications and dietary supplements.

The beneficial effects of exercise have been reliably demonstrated in research studies. Exercise can improve cardiovascular fitness, prevent obesity, and help maintain emotional well-being. With regard to cholesterol levels, increases in high density lipoprotein cholesterol (HDL) and decreases in triglyceride (TG) levels have been demonstrated consistently in people who exercise regularly. With high levels of energy expenditure, the total cholesterol level (TC) and low density lipoprotein (LDL) cholesterol levels can be positively adapted, albeit to small degrees. This improvement in the serum lipids occurs acutely after exercise as well as chronically as fitness improves and varies according to the type, intensity, and duration of exercise.

Although it is clear that some sort of physical activity is beneficial for cardiovascular health and lipid reduction, clinicians may struggle with helping patients plan their individualized lifestyle changes in physical activity. The type, frequency, duration, and intensity of exercise are topics that should be considered. This chapter discusses the benefits of certain types of exercise, discusses the considerations for certain populations when considering exercise, explains how to write an exercise

A.S. Howe
Residency Teaching Staff Physician, Director of Sports Medicine, Department of Family Medicine, Malcolm Grow Medical Center, Andrews Air Force Base, MD

B.V. Reamy (ed.), *Hyperlipidemia Management for Primary Care*,
DOI: 10.1007/978-0-387-76606-5_5, © Springer Science+Business Media, LLC 2008

prescription for an individual patient, and offers suggestions for counseling patients to begin adding increasing amounts of activity to their life.

Exercise Effects

Exercise is frequently recommended as an initial or adjunctive treatment to lower elevated cholesterol levels. Certain portions of serum lipids appear to be more sensitive to changes in a person's exercise routine. As little as a single exercise session can affect a person's lipids. Acute increases in the HDL level and reductions in TG levels can be seen within hours of an exercise session [7]. Maximum TG effects occur 18 to 24 h after the exercise session, and positive effects can persist for as long as 72 h [8,9]. This effect is most impressive in patients with elevated baseline TG levels and does not appear to require a certain threshold of exertion to occur [8].

The greatest and most consistent effect seen with exercise is an increase in HDL levels. Increases of 4% to 43% have been demonstrated after moderate exercise routines [6,9]. Endurance athletes have been studied extensively and demonstrate HDL levels 40% to 50% higher than their sedentary counterparts. The HDL increase is more than just an acute effect. As regular exercise occurs over time, aerobic fitness tends to improve. Increases in energy expenditure lead to increased HDL levels by 2 to 8 mg/dl in a dose-dependent fashion [9,10].

When combined with a moderate weight loss, low-fat diet, exercise has been shown to enhance lipid-lowering effects [11]. Exercise causes increased lipoprotein lipase and decreased hepatic lipase levels, which lead to catabolism of TG and resultant decrease in TG and increase in HDL [12].

Endurance Sports

Athletes who engage in endurance sports have consistently shown improved serum lipid profiles when compared to sedentary controls. The most consistent of these changes is in the form of an increased HDL. Multiple studies of endurance athletes compared with their sedentary counterparts demonstrate 40% to 50% higher HDL levels and 20% lower triglyceride levels [3,7,13,14]. Even mild to moderate levels of exercise have been shown to improve cholesterol levels [3].

The intensity of exercise is less important than the amount of exercise a person performs. This consideration is particularly significant when endurance exercisers are compared to sedentary controls. In a randomized, controlled trial, the effect of exercise intensity and overall amount of exercise were examined. The authors noticed an improvement in serum lipid levels in all the exercising participants when compared with the control group. The plasma levels of LDL, HDL, TG, and very low density lipoprotein (VLDL) were subfractionated such that in a typical lipid panel commonly used today only the HDL and TG levels would have shown improvement. By subfractionating, the authors could show a decreased concentration of small LDL and an increase in the average LDL size without a change in the plasma LDL total level. The intensity of exercise did not demonstrate significant improvement in regards to serum lipid levels but did improve the subject's overall fitness as measured by their VO$_2$ max [13].

A meta-analysis of studies evaluating greater than 8 weeks of aerobic exercise in men and its effects on the standard lipid profile was accomplished. The authors were able to conclude that exercise can produce statistically significant reductions in total cholesterol (TC) by 2% and TG by 9%. It also raised HDL by 3%. A statistical trend of lower LDL with exercise was noted. Despite the fact that the triglyceride levels improved by the greatest margin, it is suspected that the HDL increase and TC reduction confer the greatest benefit to an individual patient. Reducing HDL levels by 1% can increase the risk of coronary artery disease (CAD) by 2% to 3%. Similarly, a decrease in TC of only 1% has shown a 2% reduction in CAD risk [15].

Weight Training

Compared to endurance training, which results in primarily aerobic fitness, weight lifting uses primarily anaerobic metabolism. In a small study looking at sedentary men and women in their second or third decade of life, it was found that completing a progressive resistance weight training routine for 16 weeks improved the cholesterol panel by decreasing TC and LDL significantly and increasing HDL minimally. In this study, there was a significant reduction in triglycerides for women but not for men [16]. Most studies of resistance activity, such as weight training, have shown less benefit than seen with endurance programs or aerobic exercise.

Exercise Dose

It has been hypothesized that there may be an exercise threshold above which HDL levels begin to rise. However, this point has not been demonstrated. Rather, there appears to be a linear dose–response relationship between miles of walking or jogging per week and an increase in HDL levels [10].

In contrast to HDL, there may exist a specific threshold at which the LDL particle sizes change for the better. With 17–18 miles per week (27.2–28.8 km) of exercise at moderate jogging intensity, the average size of LDL particles increased [13]. A standard serum lipid panel would not have demonstrated this change in LDL, but it was elicited by examining subfractions of the LDL portion of the panel. At this exercise amount and intensity, improvement was seen in HDL and TG as well.

Specific Populations

Women

The benefit of exercise on bone health for women has been clearly established. Weight-bearing exercise increases bone mineral density and therefore reduces risk of osteoporosis [17]. The effect of exercise on serum lipids of women has also been evaluated.

It is important to consider women in two major groups when concerned about cardiovascular risk: premenopausal and postmenopausal. Menopausal transition is marked by cessation of ovarian function and resultant decrease in sex hormone levels, which translates to adverse lipid changes and a higher risk of cardiovascular disease [18]. Premenopausal athletic women have more favorable HDL, LDL, TG, and TC levels than postmenopausal athletes [17]. There may be an increased risk of CAD in formerly athletic postmenopausal women as their lipid profiles tend to be less favorable than nonathlete sedentary controls [18].

Completion of 1 year of exercise in obese and overweight previously sedentary postmenopausal women did not demonstrate significant changes in the lipid panel. On average, serum lipids were borderline elevated at the start of the study and the exercising women expended 900 kcal per week. Despite improvements in total and abdominal body fat and overall fitness level, serum lipids did not change in the women who underwent the cardiovascular exercise portion of the study [19]. Positive effects of exercise alone on the lipid panel have been observed in leaner postmenopausal women with more favorable serum lipids at baseline [20]. It has been suggested that perhaps 2 years of a more frequent exercise routine may be required to demonstrate significant lipid improvements in postmenopausal overweight and obese women [21]. Possible, too, is the need to obtain a threshold calorie burning level before lipid changes are evident. A calorie expenditure of 1200–1600 kcal/week is proposed to be necessary to see changes [22].

Lipid benefits from exercise are likely to be more prevalent in the active premenopausal population. However, given the increased CVD risk in postmenopausal women, it is clear that interventions are necessary in this population to alter risk. It seems apparent that exercise alone does not offer enough benefit in postmenopausal women and therefore should be used as adjunctive treatment with other lifestyle and medication treatments.

Children

Children and adolescents tend to participate in both spontaneous exercise and organized exercise through sports teams. Comparisons made between age- and gender-matched adolescent athletes and controls showed relatively equivalent lipid panels despite the increased organized exercise in the athlete population [23]. It appears that the relationship between training volume and serum lipids in youth is insignificant [24].

In adolescent runners, HDL levels tend to be equal in males and females younger than 14 years of age. After 14 years of age, HDL levels tend to decline across gender, but the change is larger in males [23]. This lowering of HDL is not significantly attenuated in adolescent athletes versus their age-matched controls. Pubertal changes, such as increase in adipose tissue, likely account for the lowering of HDL levels as adolescents age.

Given the foregoing observations, exercise should be considered as treatment of youth with poor serum lipid profiles. Ensuring regular cardiovascular exercise is important in youth of all ages with dyslipidemia, but evaluation of environmental and genetic factors must also occur.

Older Adults

Large clinical trials have demonstrated that treatment of elderly individuals with known CVD using lifestyle changes (exercise and diet) and drug therapy has resulted in significant reductions in cardiac morbidity and mortality [25]. Absolute risk of coronary disease increases with age in both men and women [26].

Exercise has not typically been a significant portion of hyperlipidemia treatment in elderly patients, largely because elderly individuals often do not have the capability of performing the quantity of exercise sufficient to improve serum lipids. Healthcare providers may be worried that exercise will precipitate a cardiovascular event or a fall. Given that exercise has been shown to improve conditioning and life span in the elderly, we recommend that an individualized exercise program be created for elderly patients in the setting of hyperlipidemia.

Older adults with athletic backgrounds should be encouraged to continue to maintain an age-appropriate fitness level. Former athletes who maintain age-matched fitness levels have more favorable lipid panels compared to those who become sedentary or sedentary nonathlete older adults. These same active former athletes have lower risk of coronary artery disease and improved body fat and body mass index parameters [27].

Acute Versus Chronic Effect of Exercise

Acute and chronic levels of exercise can affect serum lipids. A single exercise event has been shown to reduce triglycerides and increase high density lipoprotein (HDL) acutely [7]. This effect tends to dissipate rapidly after the exertion has ended. The beneficial change in serum lipids tends to diminish with subsequent exercise sessions. However, increasing the amount of exercise that occurs at each session does seem to increase the effect. It should be noted that this effect has been linked primarily to moderate- to high-intensity exercise sessions undertaken by trained athletes and may be more exercise than the typical untrained athlete is capable of completing [7].

The acute effect on HDL levels ranges from 4% to 43% following a single exercise session. It is unknown how long and how hard a patient must exercise to achieve maximum effect, but in trained athletes calorie expenditure as low as 350–400 kcal during a session has demonstrated benefit [7,14]. The amount of exercise as well as the duration of exercise are linked to improvements seen in cholesterol panels.

Exercise Prescriptions

Exercise prescriptions and programs have been used for years as recommendations for the improvement of physical fitness. However, similar to many lifestyle
modifications, they have met with limited success when given to unwilling patients
who demonstrate continuation at the 1-year mark of only about 50% [28]. Supervi-
sion, repetitive encouragement, frequent reassessment, achievable goal setting, and
obvious rewards may be beneficial in establishing an exercise program.

Although the primary reason for exercise prescription is to increase cardiorespiratory and flexibility fitness, it can be a powerful adjunct to therapeutic lifestyle
changes in the treatment of lipid disorders. The fitness principles of frequency, intensity, mode, and duration (otherwise known as the FITT principles for Frequency,
Intensity, Type, and Time) specify at each progressive level how the exercise
prescription *overload* (see following) will take place [29]. The primary mode used to
improve lipid panels is cardiorespiratory exercise. Thus, the majority of this section
focuses on prescribing programs with a goal of improving cardiovascular fitness.

Two Principles of Training Progression

Overload

One cannot simply begin at the endstate of the fitness goals described in the
summary of fitness goals at the end of this chapter. Any attempt to do so would
likely lead to program failure, injury, or death. A slow progression of no more than
a 5% increase in intensity or 5 min per day increase in time each week will help
avoid injury while allowing the body and mind to adapt to the increasing stresses
associated with progressive exercise programs. This slow progression is referred to
as overload. For a tissue or muscle to improve function, it must be progressively
exposed to higher stresses than it is typically exposed. After repeated exposures, the
tissue adapts and improves function [29].

Specificity

The exercise performed dictates which specific muscle groups are overloaded. Thus,
a cyclist and a swimmer have limited crossover of involved peripheral muscle
groups, whereas the cardiac effects of training benefit both activities [30]. Athletes
wishing to improve one activity (e.g., running) should focus training in that area
following the principle of specificity. However, those wishing to have a more well
rounded fitness level should vary aerobic exercise among several different cardiorespiratory activities. For the most part, those wishing to positively affect their lipid
levels should focus their training on aerobic activities. Activities dedicated toward
resistance and flexibility training serve as an adjunct to the prescribed aerobic conditioning program.

Training Session Organization

Warm-Up

As the individual transitions from rest to their exercise activity, he/she must set the conditions for his/her body to accommodate the future stresses placed on it. Light aerobic activity and gentle stretching helps facilitate this transition by loosening up the muscle groups involved, improving blood flow, and allowing the gradual mental transition to desired level of physical effort [31]. Warming up may reduce the risk of musculoskeletal injury and decrease the risk of myocardial adverse events [29]. A typical warm-up session for a runner may involve slow walking, then fast walking, and finally slow running for a total of 5 to 10 min, followed by an equal amount of time stretching the muscle groups involved in the follow-on exercise activities. Although definitive studies supporting stretching before and/or after exercise are lacking, it is generally regarded as useful for injury prevention in most populations [29].

Stimulus or Conditioning Phase

This phase is "the work-out" phase in which the exerciser seeks to improve their conditioning for whatever "event" they are training. The event may be cardiorespiratory, resistance, flexibility, or all three areas of fitness. For those seeking to make substantial improvements in lipid levels, the focus during this phase should be on large muscle group aerobic activity, such as running, cycling, swimming, or elliptical training [29].

Recreational Activities

Following the conditioning phase, or sometimes as the entire conditioning phase, a period of fun recreational games may be added to further the calorie-burning time for some aerobic exercise sessions. Example activities include Frisbee-football, running-golf (may need to coordinate having the first tee-time), nonstop volleyball, soccer, and basketball. Essentially, modification of any game to make it more nonstop in nature as well as involvement of large muscle groups extends the conditioning phase [29,32].

Cool-Down

A cool-down period is critical to returning the body to its preexercise state. This phase usually involves 5 min of decreasing intensity exercise such as slow running and then walking followed by another 5 min of stretching and other relaxation activities such as meditation or yoga [29]. This process can prevent exercise-associated collapse (EAC), which can be associated with a sudden cessation of vigorous exercise. EAC results from sudden peripheral blood pooling and resultant hypotension [33]. An initial manifestation of this condition is usually dizziness, but shortness of breath or myocardial ischemia may be the initial presentation in susceptible individuals. An adequate cool-down also serves to enhance removal of lactic acid and other metabolic waste products that lead to postexercise muscle soreness [29].

Estimating Levels of Exercise Intensity

The final exercise intensity goal for promoting lipid lowering is to exercise between 40% and 70% using the oxygen uptake reserve (VO2R), heart rate reserve (HRR), or rating of perceived exertion (RPE) methods. All three of these methods are described in this section. An initial intensity of 40% may be needed in untrained individuals to prevent orthopedic injuries and other adverse events. However, intensity levels approaching 85% may be needed to achieve lipid-lowering goals before entering the maintenance phase described in this section. Exercise intensity monitoring allows the individual to better attain the desired intensity level and allows the exercise prescribing provider to evaluate the fitness progress of the individual.

VO2 Reserve (VO2R)

The VO2R method is closely estimated by the HRR method and is difficult to use except through the use of expensive equipment, highly trained exercise testing personnel, and complicated equations. Because of this, the VO2R method is beyond the scope of this book and is reserved for the exercise specialist. Further information on this topic can be obtained from the *ACSM's Guidelines for Exercise Testing and Prescription* and its accompanying *Resource Manual* for those special situations in which these resources are available. See the Key Suggested Readings at the end of this chapter.

Heart Rate Reserve (HRR)

An essential element of the HRR* method is determining the maximum attainable heart rate (HR_{max}) for an individual. The most accurate measurement of HR_{max} is by conducting a progressive maximum exercise test, which is specific to the exercise used to achieve this maximum effort. So, depending on the exercise restrictions of the individual, the form of exercise most likely to be used for the exercise prescription should also be used to determine the maximum heart rate (HR_{max}).

---

*Heart Rate Reserve (HRR): The range of heart rate values between maximum and resting heart rates. The reserve corresponds very closely to the VO2 range from resting to maximum. %HRR reserve thus is a very good estimate of % VO2max.

If performing this assessment is not practicable or necessary in the provider's opinion, one of many estimation formulas may be used to approximate the HR_{max}. The best known formula is this:

$$HR_{max} = 220 - age$$

where "age" represents the actual age of the individual being prescribed the exercise prescription. So, for an individual age 30, this would be $HR_{max} = 220 - 30 = 190$. The variability of this method may under- or overestimate the HR_{max} by up to 10 to 12 beats/min, depending on the exact age of the individual [29]. Numerous other complex formulas have been proposed to minimize these variations, and some are more accurate than others. A meta-analysis in 2001 developed one well accepted modification to this calculation, although this equation still had a variance of 7 to 11 beats/min [34]:

$$HR_{max} = 208 - (0.7 \times age)$$

Using our 30-year-old individual, this would equate to a $HR_{max} = 208 - (0.7 \times 30) = 187$, which demonstrates a 3 beat/min difference from the previous formula.

The HRR method, a popular way of determining target heart rates for varying levels of exertion, was originally described by Karvonen et al. in 1957 [35]. The base equation follows:

$$\text{Target heart tate} = [(HR_{max} - HR_{rest}) \times \text{percent intensity}] + HR_{rest}$$

where HR_{max} is the maximum heart rate previously discussed, the HR_{rest} is the resting heart rate, and percent intensity is either the upper or lower limit of the prescribed intensity level. Using our lipid-lowering goal intensities of 40% to 70% for a 30-year-old individual and a resting heart rate of 60, it would look like this:

Target heart rate (40) = ([187–60] × 0.40) + 60 = 110.8, or roughly 111

Target heart rate (70) = ([187–60] × 0.70) + 60 = 148.9, or roughly 149

Thus, the training heart rate range for this 30-year-old would be about 111 to 149 beats/min. Unless a true progressive maximum exercise test HR_{max} is determined, a calculated HR_{max} may have up to a 12 beat/min error associated with it for all calculations made in the foregoing equations, but it is a safe and reasonable place to start in the development of an exercise prescription.

Finally, the easiest way to continuously monitor the individual's heart rate is with a heart rate monitor. Although these typically cost around $60, the price can range from $10 to several hundred dollars, depending on the capabilities of the monitor system [36]. Other alternatives include using embedded heart rate monitors in exercise equipment and self-palpating the radial artery pulse to determine the number of heart beats per minute. Because of its relative simplicity, the HRR method is the method of choice for prescribing cardiorespiratory exercise prescriptions.

Rating of Perceived Exertion (RPE)

The RPE can approximate the exercising individual's heart rate and exercise effort. However, large interindividual variability dictates that its use in monitoring exercising individuals be done with caution [29,37]. One's self-rated perception of exertion is a subjective measurement, and it can be influenced by numerous factors such as mental fatigue, environment, pain, and unfamiliar exercise modes.

A popular scale used to determine RPE is Borg's RPE Scale. This scale takes into account the exerciser's self-perceived exercise intensity, effort, and fatigue [38]. The Borg Category Scale rates exertion from 6 to 20, correlating from "very, very light" to "very, very hard." The Borg Category-Ratio Scale rates exertion from 0 to 11, corresponding from "nothing at all" to "absolute maximum" [29]. Gunnar Borg first conceived of perceived exertion in the late 1950s and has since published several books on the topic [39]. These books are excellent sources for anyone wishing to use RPE in an exercise prescription, particularly *Borg's Perceived Exertion and Pain Scales* [40].

Training Progression

Cardiorespiratory Exercise Prescription

Initial Conditioning Stage

The goal of the initial conditioning stage is to introduce the person to regular physical exercise and to promote exercise adherence. The frequency of exercise sessions during this stage is 3 to 4 times per week. This stage begins with light exercise and may slowly advance toward moderate-intensity exercise (40%–60% of HHR or VO2R), which results in minimal muscle soreness after each workout. This stage will have a variable length depending on the initial fitness level of the participant and his/her motivation toward achieving his/her fitness goals. Young, healthy individuals may move out of this stage in as little as a week, while older individuals with more health issues may be at this stage for 1 to 2 months. Typical programs include a 10- to 15-min warm-up, 15 to 20 min of aerobic conditioning, which progresses to 30 min at the end of this stage, and a 10- to 15-min cool-down [29].

Improvement Stage

During this stage, there is an attempt to reach the person's final physical fitness and lipid-lowering goals. For the goal to be accomplished, a gradual increase in the overload conditions at a more rapid pace than the initial stage will be used to achieve the desired effects. Again, the length of this stage is variable and may last 4 to 8 months depending on the individual's exercise experience, age, health status, and initial conditioning level. The intensity level will gradually increase from 50% to 70% of HHR or VO2R. Some may even vigorously increase their intensity up to nearly 85% if this intensity of exercise is needed to meet their goals. The duration of exercise should not be increased beyond 5 min per day per week; this will help avoid injury. Initial goals of increasing the frequency to 3 to 5 days per week and the duration to 35 to 40 min of cardiorespiratory exercise per session should be accomplished before any changes in intensity. Finally, small, 5% increases in intensity levels (changes in HRR or VO2R) every six or so exercise sessions will complete this stage at or above the 70% HRR or VO2R level. This stage ends when the individual reaches his/her lipid-lowering goal or his/her lipid levels plateau after the individual reaches the upper limit of tolerable training progression [29].

Maintenance Stage

Once the individual reaches his/her lipid-lowering goals or maximizes the effects from exercise, he/she enters this stage. The goal now becomes maintaining his/her current lipid levels through exercise. The exercise guidelines found in Table 5.1 should serve to meet this end [29]. Intermittently, the individual may return to the improvement stage to meet new lipid-lowering goals or to overcome potential setbacks from noncompliance with the exercise prescription. See Table 5.2 for a summary of these recommendations on cardiorespiratory training.

Resistance Exercise Prescription

The research to support the use of resistance exercise to promote weight loss and lipid lowering is less consistent, but some studies demonstrate decreases in LDL and TGs and increases in HDL with weight training. During equal times of cardiorespiratory and resistance training, resistance training burns less than half the number of calories of cardiorespiratory training [29]. Therefore, resistance training may be helpful to improve the lipid panel, but it is often not recommended as a

Table 5.1 Exercise guidelines

- Primary mode should be large muscle group aerobic activity.
- Intensity between 40% and 70% of VO2R or heart rate reserve (HRR) including rating of perceived exertion (RPE) methods.
- Frequency of 5 or more days per week to maximize caloric expenditure.
- Duration of 40–60 min (or two sessions per day of 20–30 min).
- Consistent with recommendations for long-term weight control (e.g., 200–300 min/week, 2000 kcal or more per week).

HRR, difference between maximum and resting heart rates.
Source: Data from Whaley MH, Brubaker PH, Otto RM. ACSM's guidelines for exercise testing and prescription, 7th edn. Philadelphia: Lippincott Williams & Wilkins, 2006:212; and from American College of Sports Medicine. Position Stand: appropriate intervention strategies for weight loss and prevention of weight regain for adults. Med Sci Sports Exerc 2001;33:2145–2156.

Table 5.2 Sample 6-month training progression program

Conditioning state	Week	Frequency (sessions/week)	Intensity (%HRR)	Duration (min)
Initial	1	3	40–50	15–20
	2	3–4	40–50	20–25
	3	3–4	40–60	20–25
	4	3–4	40–60	25–30
Improvement	5–7	3–4	40–65	30–35
	8–10	3–4	40–70	30–35
	11–13	4–5	40–70	35–40
	14–16	4–5	40–75	35–40
	17–20	4–5	40–75	40–50
	21–24	5	40–85	40–60
Maintenance	24+	5+	40–70	40–60

HRR, difference between maximum and resting heart rates. HRR correlates closely to VO_2 max levels from resting to maximum; therefore, %HRR approximates %VO_{2max}.
Source: Adapted with permission from Whaley MH, Brubaker PH, Otto RM. ACSM's guidelines for exercise testing and prescription, 7th edn. Philadelphia: Lippincott Williams & Wilkins, 2006:149.

primary mode for lipid lowering as endurance training is more likely to produce the desired effect. Resistance training should be used as an adjunct to promote muscular strength and endurance as part of a global health fitness program.

Modes of resistance training include free weights, machines, resistance bands, exercise balls, and personal body weight or partner resisted exercises. Any of these modes may provide excellent resistance training if performed correctly using proper techniques, utilizing proper rest, and using adequate concentric (muscle shortening) and eccentric (muscle lengthening) resistance. Resistance training should involve all the major muscle groups: back, chest, shoulders, arms, abdominals, hips, thighs, and legs [29].

Healthy individuals benefit from as little as one set of 3 to 20 reps done to volitional fatigue (muscle failure or a RPE of 19 to 20). Individuals with moderate to high cardiovascular risk should limit their resistance training to 2 to 3 reps short of volitional fatigue (RPE of 15 to 16); this will decrease the catecholamine response to resistance training and limit the risk of adverse events. Each major muscle group should be exercised on 2 to 3 nonconsecutive days per week. See Table 5.3 for a summary of these recommendations on resistance training.

Flexibility Exercise Prescription

There is no current literature that supports the use of flexibility training in lowering lipid levels or for weight loss. However, flexibility training as part of a global health fitness program is recommended by a number of organizations, including the American College of Sports Medicine.

Stretching programs should involve the static stretching of all the major muscle groups and be performed a minimum of 2 to 3 days per week (ideally, almost all days of the week). Ballistic stretching has been implicated as a risk factor for muscle

Table 5.3 Summary of endstate exercise prescription for dyslipidemia

Physical Fitness Component	Frequency	Intensity	Duration	Activity
Cardiorespiratory	5+ days/week	40%–70% VO2R or HRR (e.g., 12-14 RPE)	40–60 min/day or two 20- to 30- min sessions	Large muscle groups
Resistance	2–3 days/week	Volitional fatigue (MMF) (e.g., 19–20 RPE) Stop 2–3 reps before volitional fatigue (e.g., 16 RPE)	1 set of 3–20 repetitions	8–10 exercises Include all major Ormuscle groups
Flexibility	2–7 days/week	Stretch to tightness at the end of the range or motion but not to pain	15–30 s 2–4 times per Stretch	Static stretch all major muscle groups

Source: Adapted with permission from Whaley MH, Brubaker PH, Otto RM. ACSM's guidelines for exercise testing and prescription, 7th edn. Philadelphia: Lippincott Williams & Wilkins, 2006:206.)

strain and should be avoided [29]. However, many high-level and elite athletes routinely use dynamic stretching during their 10- to 15-min warm-up phase. All stretching programs are preceded by a warm-up or cardiorespiratory exercise period. Stretches are held at the end range of motion in a position of tightness, without pain. Each stretch is performed two to four times and held for a count of 15 to 30 s [29].

Special Considerations

Although maximal and submaximal exercise testing can be used to determine an individual's fitness level or maximal heart rate, care must be taken with proper risk stratification of potential exercisers so as to avoid adverse events. Low-risk individuals (asymptomatic men less than 45 and woman less than 55 years of age without more than one cardiac risk factor) may receive an exercise prescription without any limitations and may undergo maximal exercise testing if desired to determine the HR_{max}. Moderate- or high-risk individuals should be medically cleared before engaging in exercise testing or any vigorous exercise.

Modifications to exercise testing or considerations for exercise prescription may be required based on an individual's comorbid medical conditions (e.g., obesity, hypertension, coronary artery disease, congestive heart failure, pulmonary disease, diabetes, and/or arthritis). In general, low-risk individuals may follow an unsupervised exercise prescription, but moderate- and high-risk individuals should be supervised by appropriately trained exercise specialists commensurate with the degree of cardiorespiratory, pulmonary, or metabolic disease [29].

Finally, special mention is given to dyslipidemic individuals taking lipid-lowering medications (e.g., statins and fibrates). Potential side effects of these medications are myopathy and hepatic side effects [6]. These conditions can be initiated or worsened through exercise. Therefore, it is recommended that these conditions be screened for intermittently during office visits as the individual progresses through the training stages. Once the individual safely attains the maintenance stage of training, normal once-a-year screening is reinstituted. Those individuals on high- to maximum-dose statin therapy, on combination therapy, or with persistent or worsening muscle soreness not easily attributable to muscle overload may require laboratory screening with muscle enzyme testing (creatinine kinase or aldolase) to diagnose a serious myopathy.

Americans in Motion

The American Academy of Family Physicians (AAFP) has created a family-centered wellness program called Americans In Motion (AIM) in response to the rising overweight/obesity problem among children and adults [41]. This public health initiative concentrates on a central theme: fitness. It encourages all individuals to reach at least 10,000 steps per day. By focusing on physical activity, nutrition, and emotional well-being for each individual patient, there is a hope that the lessons taught to patients will promote healthy family living as well.

The program targets three populations: family physicians as fitness role models, the family medicine office for promoting a healthy patient care environment, and patients and the public in both the clinical and community setting. Clearly, this audience can be expanded to any provider of health care (nurse practitioners, physician assistants, athletic trainers, physical therapists, nutritionists, etc.), as the "teaching moments" regarding healthy living occur during many different patient interactions.

How to Counsel a Patient on Implementation of the AIM Program

The purpose of the AIM program is to encourage and support family physicians to address the problem of obesity and decreasing activity levels present in our society today. In a survey by the American Academy of Family Physicians, it was found that 60% of physicians have a problem with their own weight. Seventy percent of the respondents reported regular exercise and that they feel like a fitness role model in society. As part of the AIM program, there is focus on the family physician as a role model of fitness and health. The AAFP encourages all their academy members to wear a pedometer to evaluate their own physical activity levels. Wearing a pedometer raises both awareness and the actual amount of daily movement. The AIM goal of 10,000 steps a day has motivated many family physicians and their office staff to increase their daily activity level.

Office staff teams are encouraged to take part in the program as well. Moving more by creating a lunchtime walking group, eating better in the office, and taking

Table 5.4 Americans In Motion (AIM) program summary

BE ACTIVE	EAT SMART	FEEL GOOD
Increase daily activity	Make healthy meal choices	Choose healthy activities that make you feel better
Take the stairs instead of elevatorPark further away and walkBegin a regular exercise program	Add fruits, vegetables, and grains to daily dietMonitor calorie intake to approximate calorie expenditure	Focus on emotional health as part of overall fitnessFocus on modeling positive behaviors rather than direct weight loss or body appearance

Source: Data from AIM brochure: www.aafp.org/aim/cmebulletin.

part in encouraging patients to make healthy changes in their lives are a few of the positive interventions offices can begin.

Teaching patients how to increase their physical activity in their daily lives focuses on creating lasting fitness changes that can be sustained over a lifetime. Simple goals, such as increasing the number of steps walked in 1 day, are the starting point for most patients. Educating patients about healthy snack ideas and meal choices, for example, including grains and fruits and vegetables into their daily diet, is a simple start on the road to more healthy eating styles. Guiding patients to consider their own emotional well-being as well as that of their family when choosing activities is encouraged as well.

Implementing the AIM program in the life of the provider, office staff, or patients can be summarized as follows: *Be Active, Eat Smart, Feel Good!*

More information is available at the AIM website: www.americansinmotion.org. and in Table 5.4.

Conclusion

Participation in regular exercise can decrease risk of atherosclerotic cardiovascular disease. In part, this occurs because of the improvement exercise produces in serum lipids. Increasing HDL-C levels and decreasing TG and TC can be anticipated by most adults who participate in a regular exercise program at least 5 days per week.

It is important to assess a patient's risk of exercising before induction of an exercise program. Patients with high cholesterol often have a history of CVD or other risk factors for CVD. This population of individuals deserves special attention focused on safety and moderation when beginning a routine. A clinician may consider an evaluation for ischemic heart disease before induction of an exercise program to determine its safety.

Exercise should be part of every patient's therapy for elevated serum lipid levels, regardless of the other treatment employed. It should be motivating to patients that even small levels of exercise have benefits in reducing lipids. Ideally, this will result in lower CVD risk to the individual. A sample exercise prescription form for use in an office setting is shown in Fig. 5.1 .

EXERCISE PRESCRIPTION

NAME_____ AGE___ RESTING HEART RATE: _____

CVD risk factors: HTN   HLP   CAD   DMII   OBESITY   FHx CAD   SMOKER

HEART RATE GOALS:

HRmax = 220 – age of patient × TARGET HR = (HRmax–HRrest)*intensity% + HR rest

EASY (40%): _____   MODERATE (70%): _____   HARD (85%): _____

TYPE	DURATION (MINUTES)	DAYS PER WEEK	INTENSITY[a]
RUNNING/JOGGING			
BRISK WALK			
BIKING			
ELLIPTICAL TRAINER			
SWIMMING			
WEIGHT TRAINING			

CLASSES:

YOGA			
PILATES			
SPINNING			
AEROBICS			

[a]**INTENSITY:** VERY EASY   EASY   MODERATE   HARD   VERY HARD

STOP EXERCISING IF YOU HAVE CHEST PAIN, BECOME SEVERELY SHORT OF
BREATH OR FEEL LIKE YOU MAY PASS OUT AND ALERT A HEALTHCARE PROVIDER

	PRE-EXERCISE	3 MONTHS	6 MONTHS	12 MONTHS
TOTAL CHOLESTEROL				
TRIGLYCERIDES				
HDL				
LDL				
WEIGHT				
BODY MASS INDEX				
BLOOD PRESSURE				

Fig. 5.1 Exercise prescription

References

1. Minino AM, Heron M, Smith B. Deaths: preliminary data for 2004. Division of Vital Statistics. National Center for Health Statistics. Current as of 12 Sep 2005. www.cdc.gov/nchs/. Last viewed 4 Nov 2006.
2. Lloyd-Jones DM, Larson MG, Beiser A, et al. Lifetime risk of developing coronary heart disease. Lancet 1999;353(9147):89–92.
3. Bhalodkar NC, Blum S, Rana T, Bhalodkar A, Kitchappa R, Enas E. Effect of leisure time exercise on high-density lipoprotein cholesterol, its subclasses, and size in Asian Indians. Am J Cardiol 2005;96:98–100.

4. Blair SN, Jackson AS. Physical fitness and activity as separate heart disease risk factors: a meta-analysis. Med Sci Sports Exerc 2001;33:762–764.
5. Stamler J, Wentworth D, Neaton JD. Is relationship between serum cholesterol and risk of premature death from coronary heart disease continuous and graded? Findings in 356,222 primary screenees of the Multiple Risk Factor Intervention Trial (MRFIT). JAMA 1986;256:2823–2828.
6. Reamy BV, Thompson PD. Lipid disorders in athletes. Curr Sports Med Rep 2004;3:70–76.
7. Thompson PD, Crouse SF, Goodpaster B, Kelley D, Moyna N, Pescatello L. The acute versus the chronic response to exercise. Med Sci Sports Exerc 2001;33(6):S438–S445.
8. Cullinane E, Siconolfi S, Saritelli A, et al. Acute decrease in serum triglycerides with exercise: is there a threshold for an exercise effect? Metabolism 1982;31:844–847.
9. MacKnight JM. Exercise considerations in hypertension, obesity and dyslipidemia. Clin Sports Med 2003;20:101–121.
10. Kokkinos PF, Holland JC, Narayan P, et al. Miles run per week and high-density lipoprotein cholesterol levels in healthy, middle-aged men: a dose–response relationship. Arch Intern Med 1995;155(4):415–420.
11. Grundy SM, Blackburn G, Higgins M, et al. Physical activity in the prevention and treatment of obesity and its comorbidities. Med Sci Sports Exerc 1999;31(suppl 1):502–508.
12. Blackburn H, Jacobs JD. Physical activity and the risk of coronary heart disease. N Engl J Med 1988;319:1217–1219.
13. Kraus WE, Houmard JA, Duscha BD, et al. Effects of the amount and intensity of exercise on plasma lipoproteins. N Engl J Med 2002;347:1483–1492.
14. Kantor MA, Cullinane EM, Sady SP, Herbert PN, Thompson PD. Exercise acutely increases HDL-cholesterol and lipoprotein lipase activity in trained and untrained men. Metabolism 1987;36:188–192.
15. Kelley GA, Kelley KS. Aerobic exercise and lipids and lipoproteins in men: a meta-analysis of randomized controlled trials. J Mens Health Gender 2006;3(1):61–70.
16. Goldberg L, Elliot DL, Schultz RW, Kloster FE. Changes in lipid and lipoprotein levels after weight training. JAMA 1984;252(4):504–506.
17. Chen KT, Yang RS. Effects of exercise on lipid metabolism and musculoskeletal fitness in female athletes. World J Gastroenterol 2004;10(1):122–126.
18. Rosano GM, Fini M. Postmenopausal women and cardiovascular risk: impact of hormone replacement therapy. Cardiol Rev 2002;10:51–60.
19. Mohanka M, Irwin M, Heckbert SR, et al. Serum lipoproteins in overweight/obese postmenopausal women: a one-year exercise trial. Med Sci Sports Exerc 2006;38(2):231–239.
20. Asikainen TM, Miilunpalo S, Kukkonen-Harjula K, et al. Walking trials in postmenopausal women: effect of low doses of exercise and exercise fractionization on coronary risk factors. Scand J Med Sci Sports 2003;13:284–292.
21. King AC, Haskell WL, Young DR, Oka RK, Stefanick ML. Long-term effects of varying intensities and formats of physical activity on participation rates, fitness, and lipoproteins in men and women aged 50–65 years. Circulation 1995;91:2596–2604.
22. Kokkinos PF, Fernhall B. Physical activity and high density lipoprotein cholesterol levels: what is the relationship? Sports Med 1999;28:307–314.
23. Eisenmann JC. Blood lipids and lipoproteins in child and adolescent athletes. Sports Med 2002;32(5):297–307.
24. Eisenmann JC, Womack CJ, Reeves MJ, et al. Blood lipids of young distance runners: distribution and inter-relationships among training volume, peak oxygen consumption, and body fatness. Eur J Appl Physiol 2001;85:104–112.
25. Miettinen TA, Pyorala K, Olsson AG, et al., for the Scandinavian Simvastatin Study Group. Cholesterol-lowering therapy in women and elderly patients with myocardial infarction or angina pectoris: findings from the Scandinavian Simvastatin Survival Study (4S). Circulation 1997;96:4211.
26. Grundy SM, Cleeman JI, Rifkind BM, Kuller LH. Cholesterol lowering in the elderly population. Coordinating Committee of the National Cholesterol Education Program. Arch Intern Med 1999;159:1670.

27. Dey SK, Ghosh C, Debray P, Chatterjee M. Coronary artery disease risk factors & their association with physical activity in older athletes. J Cardiovasc Risk 2002;9:383–392.
28. Dishman R, ed. Exercise adherence: its impact on public health. Champaign, IL: Human Kinetics, 1988:237–258.
29. Whaley M, ed. ACSM's guidelines for exercise testing and prescription, 7th edn. Philadelphia: Lippincott Williams & Wilkins, 2006.
30. Gollnick P. Effects of training on enzyme activity and fiber composition of human skeletal muscle. J Appl Physiol 1973;34:107–111.
31. Bishop D. Potential mechanisms and the effects of passive warm-up on exercise performance. Sports Med 2003;33:439–454.
32. Franklin B, Stoedefalke K. Games-as-aerobics: activities for cardiac rehabilitation programs. In: Fardy P, Franklin B, et al. (eds) Current issues in cardiac rehabilitation: training techniques in cardiac rehabilitation. Champaign, IL: Human Kinetics, 1998:106–136.
33. Brennan F, O'Conner F. Emergency triage of collapsed endurance athletes. Physician Sports Med 2005;33(3):28–36.
34. Tanaka H, Monahan K, Seals D. Age-predicted maximal heart rate revisited. J Am Coll Cardiol 2001;37:153–156.
35. Karvonen M, Kentala K, Mustala O. The effects of training on heart rate: a longitudinal study. Ann Med Exp Biol Fenn 1957;35:307–315.
36. http://amazon.com/s/ref=nb˙ss˙gw/104-6421239-8121540?url=search-alias%3Daps&field-ke ywords=heart+rate+monitor.
37. Whaley M, Brubaker P, Kaminsky L, et al. Validity of rating of perceived exertion during graded exercise testing in apparently healthy adults and cardiac patients. J Cardiopulm Rehabil 1997;17:261–267.
38. Noble B, Borg G, Jacobs I, et al. A category-ratio perceived exertion scale: relationship to blood and muscle lactates and heart rate. Med Sci Sports Exerc 1983;15:523–528.
39. https://www.hkaustralia.com/products/showproduct.cfm?isbn=0880116234.
40. Borg G. Borg's perceived exertion and pain scales. Champaign, IL: Human Kinetics, 1998.
41. Americans in Motion, public health initiative created by the American Academy of Family Physicians. www.americansinmotion.org; www.aafp.org website 4 Nov 2006.

Suggested Key Readings

ACSM Position Stand. Appropriate intervention strategies for weight loss and prevention of weight regain in adults. Med Sci Sports Exerc 2001;33:2145–2156.
ACSM Position Stand. The recommended quality and quantity of exercise for developing and maintaining cardiorespiratory and muscle fitness, and flexibility in healthy adults. Med Sci Sports Exerc 1998;30:975–991.
ACSM's Guidelines for exercise testing and prescription, 7th edn. Philadelphia: Lippincott Williams & Wilkins, 2006.
ACSM's resource manual for guidelines for exercise testing and prescription, 5th edn. Philadelphia: Lippincott Williams & Wilkins, 2005.

Chapter 6
Drug Treatment

Brian V. Reamy and Brian K. Unwin

General Principles of Drug Treatment of Hyperlipidemia

Many patients require pharmacologic therapy to reach their lipid goals in addition to the therapeutic lifestyle interventions of diet, therapeutic foods, and exercise discussed in previous chapters. The following five key principles should guide drug selection:

1. Be sure the intensity of therapy is guided by an accurate coronary risk assessment of the patient.
2. Maximize monotherapy before starting combination drug therapy.
3. Prescribe a dosage of a statin designed to reach your target LDL level as your *initial* dose as opposed to dosage titration.
4. Select medicines appropriate for any patient comorbidity.
5. Individualize your therapeutic plan for each patient by remaining cognizant of unique issues that special populations may present (see Chapter 7).

Each of these five key principles is now be reviewed in detail.

Base Intensity of Drug Therapy on an Accurate Risk Assessment

Intensity of therapy should be guided by an accurate coronary risk assessment. If a patient already has coronary disease or an equivalent, such as diabetes mellitus, peripheral arterial disease, carotid disease, or an abdominal aortic aneurysm, they are at high risk and further risk calculation is not required. The physician is employing secondary prevention, and the most intense low density lipoprotein

B.V. Reamy
Chair and Associate Professor, Department of Family Medicine, Uniformed Services University of the Health Sciences, Bethesda, MD
e-mail: breamy@usuhs.mil

B.V. Reamy (ed.), *Hyperlipidemia Management for Primary Care*,
DOI: 10.1007/978-0-387-76606-5_6, © Springer Science+Business Media, LLC 2008

(LDL) lowering and optimization of high density lipoprotein (HDL) and triglycerides (TG) is supported by the evidence.

For patients without manifest cardiovascular disease, it is important to base the intensity of therapy on a formal quantitative risk assessment. Using maximal drug therapy for a patient at low risk for a vascular event is unlikely to lead to a beneficial outcome and is very likely to be economically costly or trigger side effects. In contrast, using minimal therapy for a patient at very high risk for a coronary event is equally unsound.

The NCEP/ATP Guidelines are based on the use of a Framingham Risk assessment that can be found and downloaded at www.nhlbi.nih.gov. Other coronary risk calculators are available free of charge. A very useful one is that from the Medical College of Wisconsin at www.intmed.mcw.edu/clincalc/heartrisk.html. It is important to recognize that risk calculations need to be updated periodically for an individual patient. For example, all other values being equal, a man aging only 1 year, from 44 to 45 years of age, will triple his 10-year coronary risk from 1% to 3%. Aging or other changes in health status can significantly alter LDL treatment goals and therefore the desired intensity of drug therapy.

Maximize Monotherapy Before Starting Combination Therapy

Many patients can be controlled with a single agent. Using only one drug saves money and lessens side effects. In particular, most patients with vascular disease are already on multiple medications for other conditions: using monotherapy for hyperlipidemia helps to simplify their overall drug regimen. A corollary to the foregoing statement is that, once monotherapy is maximized, it is important to use combination therapy without hesitation if it is needed to achieve lipid targets based on an individualized patient risk assessment.

Choose an Initial Dose Potent Enough to Reach Goal LDL

It is important to initiate a dose of a statin designed to reach your LDL goal. The potency of statins is predictable based on each agent and the tablet strength (Table 6.1). Starting drug therapy with an agent and dose selected to reach your LDL target accomplishes several goals. It helps to avoid staying at a dosage that is too low, minimizing the need for return visits, lessens the cost of repeat laboratory tests, and improves compliance and satisfaction among patients. A corollary to this rule is that you get maximal lipid lowering from this initial standard dose of a statin. Each doubling of a statin dose leads to only 6% more LDL-lowering potency, commonly known as the "Rule of Sixes."

Assess Individual Patient Comorbidity

It is important to be aware of patient comorbidity in the selection and dosage of cholesterol lowering medication. Chronic liver disease, pregnancy, and a previous

Table 6.1 Initial statin dosages and percentage of low density lipoprotein (LDL) reduction

Desired % LDL reduction	Initial statin and dose/day
30% to 40%	Fluvastatin 80 mg
	Lovastatin 40 mg
	Pravastatin 40 mg
	Simvastatin 20 to 40 mg
	Atorvastatin 10 to 20 mg
40% to 50%	Simvastatin 40 to 60 mg
	Atorvastatin 20 to 40 mg
50% to 60%	Rosuvastatin 10 to 20 mg
	Atorvastatin 60 to 80 mg
More than 60%	Rosuvastatin 40 mg
	Atorvastatin 80 mg

Note: Simvastatin 80 mg is *not* included in this table. Even though it can lower LDL significantly, it has a much higher rate of rhabdomyolysis and is not considered as safe as the other statin choices.

history of rhabdomyolysis are contraindications to the use of many medications. Commonly, patients with vascular disease comorbidity may be on anticoagulation with warfarin. Most cholesterol-lowering medications affect either the absorption or metabolism of warfarin and require dosage adjustment of a patient's anticoagulant.

Special Populations May Require Unique Treatments

Special populations such as women, children, the elderly, elite athletes, and certain ethnic groups present unique issues for consideration in the prescription of drug therapy. Asian subpopulations tend to develop twice the level of serum rosuvastatin than non-Asian patients. The elderly are more likely to be on a multiple of other medications that require dosage adjustment. Children at high risk for vascular disease have been limited to the use of resins, although data are growing on the safety of statins. Women of childbearing age need to be counseled about the lack of safety of most lipid-lowering agents during gestation. Finally, elite athletes engaged in extreme sports such as ultramarathons who become severely dehydrated are more likely to have side effects and may require dose changes around competitive events. Chapter 7 reviews issues with these special populations in more detail.

Agents

There are seven main classes of lipid-lowering agents in common use. New classes are in various stages of development and are reviewed later in this chapter. These classes are resins, absorption inhibitors, niacin, fibrates, statins, fish oil, and combination agents. Tables 6.2, 6.3, 6.4, and 6.5 summarize the types, dosages, and uses of these medications.

Table 6.2 Resins and absorption inhibitors

Medication	Dosage	LDL reduction	TG reduction	HDL increase	Side effects
Resins					
Colestipol (Colestid®)	4–8 g bid	10% to 20%	May increase up to 20%	Minimal	Bloating, constipation, flatulence common
Cholestyramine (Questran®)	5–10 g bid				
Colesvelam (Welchol®)	6 capsules per day or 3 capsules bid				Interferes with absorption of many medications (less with colesvelam)
Absorption inhibitor					
Ezetimibe (Zetia®)	10 mg qd	15% to 20%	5% to 10%	1% to 3%	Minimal; occasional GI upset

HDL, high density lipoprotein; TG, triglycerides.

Table 6.3 Fibrates and niacin

Medication	Dosage	LDL reduction	TG reduction	HDL increase	Side effects
Fibrates					
Gemfibrozil (Lopid®)	600 mg bid	Minimal effect or slight increase	20% to 50%	10% to 20%	Nausea, rare hepatitis, myositis (especially with gemfibrozil + statin)
Fenofibrate (Tricore®)	48 to 148 mg po qd				
Niacin					
Short acting (Niacor®)	500–1500 mg bid	10% to 25% (dose dependent)	20% to 50%	15% to 35%	Flushing, nausea, dyspepsia, pruritus, rash, hepatitis, glucose intolerance, gout
Extended release (Niaspan®)	500–2000 mg at h.s.				

Resins or Bile Acid Sequestrants

Three bile acid sequestrants are available: cholestyramine (Questran®) and many other trade names), colestipol (Colestid®), and colesevelam (Welchol®). These drugs bind to cholesterol in the gut and are not absorbed from the gastrointestinal tract, which makes them very safe. Each can lower LDL cholesterol as much as 20%. In patients with hypertriglyceridemia, they can elevate triglycerides further [1].

Dosage and Actions

Cholestyramine is supplied as packets of powder or granules for mixing with water or juice for oral consumption at a dosage of 8 g per day divided into two to three

Table 6.4 Statins

Medication	Dosage[a]	LDL reduction	TG reduction	HDL increase	Side effects
Atorvastatin (Lipitor®)	10 to 80 mg qd	35% to 65%	15% to 40%	5% to 10%	Myalgias, hepatitis, rhabdomyolysis (rare)
Fluvastatin (Lescol®)	20 to 80 mg qd	15% to 35%	10% to 20%	3% to 7%	Same
Lovastatin (Mevacor®)	20 to 40 mg qd	20% to 35%	5% to 10%	5%	Same
Pravastatin[b] (Pravachol®)	10 to 40 mg qd	20% to 40%	10% to 25%	3% to 10%	Same
Rosuvastatin[c] (Crestor®)	5 to 40 mg qd	40% to 70%	10% to 30%	5% to 15%	Same
Simvastatin (Zocor®)	10 to 60 mg qd	25% to 50%	10% to 25%	5% to 10%	Same

[a]Although higher doses of some statins are FDA approved, they are either ineffective (lovastatin and pravastatin at 80 mg qd) or have a much greater risk of myositis (simvastatin 80 mg qd).
[b]Pravastatin has a lower rate of drug interactions and side effects because of a dual pathway of elimination.
[c]Rosuvastin has a higher rate of myositis in Asians.

Table 6.5 Fish oil and combination agents

Medication	Dosage	LDL reduction	TG reduction	HDL increase	Side effects
Combination agents					
Ezetimibe + simvastatin (Vytorin®)	10 mg + 10, 20, 40, or 80 mg simvastatin	Up to 60%	10% to 25%	5% to 10%	Myalgias, hepatitis, myositis
Niacin + lovastatin (Advicor®)	500/20 mg 1000/20 mg	Up to 45%	Up to 40%	Up to 40%	Flushing, hepatitis
Fish oil					
OTC	3 to 15 g total/day	Minimal	5% to 50%	Minimal	Fishy taste, belching, fishy
Omacor®[a]	3 to 12 g total/day	Minimal	20% to 50%	Minimal	sweat, diarrhea, weight gain

[a]Omacor® may have fewer side effects than OTC fish oil.

doses per day. It is typically dosed just before a meal. Colestipol is supplied as tablets or granules for mixing with water or juice for oral consumption at a dosage of 10 g per day divided into two or three doses. It is also dosed before a meal. Colesevalam is dosed at 3.75 g per day given in one or two doses before a meal.

Adverse Effects

The side effects of cholestyramine and colestipol are similar. Most patients are troubled by bloating, constipation, nausea, and eructation. These symptoms can lessen over time in patients who are able to continue the drugs for several months. They also block the absorption of many other medications, so caution should be exercised when they are added to a previously stable drug regimen. Anticoagulant blood levels are a particular problem. Colesevalem has slightly fewer side effects and drug interactions than cholestyramine and colestipol.

Usage

Resins are primarily used to lower LDL cholesterol. Given their side effects, this is usually as an adjunct to other lipid-lowering therapy. Patients with diarrhea-predominate irritable bowel syndrome (IBS) can benefit from resins as part of their lipid-lowering regimen. The constipating side effect can have a therapeutic effect in patients with IBS.

Absorption Inhibitors

At present, the only U.S. Food and Drug Administration (FDA)-approved member of this class is ezetimibe (Zetia®). It was released in 2003. Several other members of this class are currently in development.

Dosage and Actions

Ezetimibe is available in a 10-mg tablet and is dosed once daily with or without food. Ezetimibe selectively inhibits intestinal absorption of dietary and biliary cholesterol in the small intestine. It is then excreted in the stool. It lowers LDL 17%, TG by 6%, and increases HDL by 1.3% [2]. It can be combined with a statin to increase the intensity of LDL lowering.

Adverse Effects

Ezetimibe is generally very well tolerated. Transaminase elevations can rarely occur and are more likely if the medication is used in combination with a statin. Because ezetimibe increases cholesterol concentration in bile, it theoretically could trigger gallbladder disease.

Usage

Ezetimibe is primarily used for LDL lowering as an adjunct to other forms of LDL-lowering therapy. Patients with severe side effects to other lipid-lowering drugs rarely have side effects from ezetimibe. However, outcome studies on the use of ezetimibe monotherapy for the prevention of atherosclerotic vascular disease are lacking.

Niacin

Niacin, or nicotinic acid, affects all portions of the lipid profile in a beneficial fashion. It lowers LDL, lowers TG, and raises HDL. Formulations of niacin range from over-the-counter (OTC) nutritional supplements to prescription tablets designed for immediate release to long-acting and extended release formulations. Each formulation is designed to lessen the common side effects that frequently occur with the use of niacin.

Dosage and Actions

Niacin works primarily by inhibiting the production of very low density lipoprotein (VLDL) particles in the liver. It increases HDL more than any other drug currently on the market [1]. It also decreases TG and changes LDL from small and more dense particles to larger and less dense forms. Lower doses of niacin, from 500 to 1500 mg per day, primarily affect HDL and TG whereas higher doses, up to 3000 mg per day, may be required for significant LDL lowering as well. Immediate-release niacin is available over the counter or by prescription (Niacor®) and requires two to three time per day dosing. Older, long-acting niacin is a prescription medication that has a much higher rate of liver side effects compared to other formulations and should no longer be used [3]. Extended-release niacin (Niaspan®) can be dosed once daily and has the lowest rate of side effects of any niacin formulation. It is dosed from 500 to 2000 mg per day.

Adverse Effects

Niacin causes side effects in more than 50% of patients, frequently enough to severely limit its practical use in clinical medicine. These side effects can include skin flushing, pruritus, or cholinergic urticaria. Gastrointestinal cramping and dyspepsia are also common. Dry eyes, glucose intolerance (including a minor worsening of glucose control in diabetics), hyperuricemia, hepatitis, and acanthosis nigricans are less common but serious side effects. In patients with diabetes, the minor deterioration in glucose control is thought to be worth the benefit of the control of hyperlipidemia and should not limit the use of niacin in patients with diabetes. Rather, it is important to monitor glucose and adjust the intensity of diabetes treatment when initiating niacin. Gouty arthritis is thought to be a contraindication to therapy with niacin.

Side effects tend to decrease with long-term use and can be minimized by a slow dosage titration, pretreatment with 81 to 325 mg aspirin 30 min before taking niacin, and avoiding the consumption of niacin on an empty stomach. It is also significant that many patients can take lower doses of niacin without side effects (500–1000 mg) but have significant side effects at doses greater than 1000 mg per day. Thus, niacin is a medication that can be used as part of a combination therapy even if side effects limit its usefulness as monotherapy.

Usage

Niacin is currently the most potent agent available to raise HDL. It is also used to lower TG. Side effects limit its usage at high doses (greater then 1000 mg per day) for LDL lowering. It can be a very useful adjunctive medication for combination therapy in patients on statins who require more reduction of TG and elevation of HDL.

Fibrate

Fibric acid derivatives or fibrates are available in two formulations in the United States, gemfibrozil (Lopid®) and fenofibrate (Tricor®). Benzafibrate and clofibrate are available in other parts of the world.

Dosage and Actions

Gemfibrozil is dosed at 600 mg twice per day. Fenofibrate has been recently reformulated and is dosed at either 48 mg once per day or 145 mg once per day. These drugs are used primarily to lower TG and raise HDL. Fibrates may cause an elevation in LDL cholesterol, although they tend to shift the form of LDL from a more dense to a less dense and less atherogenic particle size. All fibrates are agonists of perioxisome proliferators activated receptor-α (PPAR-α), where they upregulate lipoprotein lipase and apolipoprotein A-1 genes, leading to a reduction in TG and an increase of HDL.

Adverse Effects

Fibrates can sometimes lead to nausea, hepatitis, myositis, and cholelithiasis. A transaminitis may occur in 2% of patients, but symptomatic hepatitis is much rarer [1]. They can also interact with statins to increase the risk of rhabdomyolysis. Recently, it has become clear that this drug interaction is primarily limited to gemfibrozil and is unlikely to occur with fenofibrate. Most experts believe that fenofibrate is the *only* fibrate that should be combined with a statin when this combination is needed to reach a lipid goal.

Usage

Fibrates are primarily used to lower triglycerides and raise HDL cholesterol. They are used as monotherapy or in combination therapy with statins in patients with combined hyperlipidemia. Fibrates are particularly useful in patients with diabetes or metabolic syndrome because hypertriglyceridemia and low HDL are very common in these syndromes.

Statins

HMG-CoA reductase inhibitors or statins have become the workhorses of drug therapy for hyperlipidemia because of their efficacy at decreasing atherogenic

LDL, their low rate of side effects, and the abundance of disease-oriented and patient-oriented evidence supporting their utility. At present, six statins are available in the United States: atorvastatin (Lipitor®), fluvastatin (Lescol®), lovastatin (Mevacor®), pravastatin (Pravacol®), rosuvastatin (Crestor®), and simvastatin (Zocor®). As of 2006, both lovastatin and simvastatin were available in generic formulations.

Dosage and Actions

The doses of each statin are reviewed in Tables 6.1 and 6.4. The potency of each statin is predictable in its ability to lower LDL. Therefore, it is important to pick the correct statin at the correct dose to achieve the degree of LDL lowering desired. In general, statins can be divided into three groups: low potency (fluvastatin), medium potency (lovastatin and pravastatin), and high potency (atorvastatin, rosuvastatin, and simvastatin). HMG-CoA reductase is the enzyme that catalyzes the rate-limiting step in cholesterol synthesis. Statins are potent inhibitors of this enzyme, which leads to a reduction in free cholesterol in hepatocytes, triggering a secondary increase in the expression of LDL receptors. This receptor upregulation leads to a further reduction of cholesterol. The full upregulation typically occurs in 6 weeks but can require up to 12 weeks. Therefore, the full potency of statins is not realized in some patients until 12 weeks after their initiation.

In addition to decreasing LDL cholesterol from 20% to 60%, all statins raise HDL to a small degree, from 3% to 15%. This effect is most pronounced with rosuvastatin. In addition, atorvastatin seems to have the greatest concomitant effect on decreasing triglycerides. All statins should be preferentially dosed in the evening or at bedtime. They are approximately 10% more potent when dosed in the evening for patients who sleep at night. Most hepatic production of cholesterol occurs from 2 A.M. to 3 A.M., which is the time that an evening dose of a statin will have its peak serum level. The opposite effect is true for patients who sleep during the daytime hours.

Statins also exert a multitude of other metabolic effects that are generally classified as antiinflammatory. These effects are so numerous and varied that they have been termed the "beneficial pleiotropic effects" of statins. These antiinflammatory effects are what have led to many off-label uses of statins for autoimmune conditions and inflammatory syndromes such as rheumatoid arthritis.

Adverse Effects

Muscle pain, myopathy, and increased liver enzymes are the main potential side effects from statins. Myalgias may occur in 5% to 10% of patients taking statins for reasons that are still unclear. Rhabdomyolysis is extremely rare, occurring in fewer than 1 per 10 million prescriptions [4–6]. Rhabdomyolysis can be prevented by the prompt discontinuation of the agent when muscle pain and elevated muscle enzymes (creatine kinase or aldolase) occur. Unexplained muscle pain should prompt investigation for myopathy; however, the routine monitoring of muscle enzymes is not supported by any evidence. The risk and severity of severe myopathy is increased in patients with hepatic dysfunction, renal failure, or severe congestive heart failure.

An increase of serum aminotransferase levels occurs in 0.5% to 2.0% of patients taking statins [6]. This hepatic side effect is dose dependent. Symptomatic hepatitis is rare, and discontinuation of the statin is not required until the transaminases are more than three times normal. It is advisable to check liver function tests at baseline, after 12 weeks of therapy, and annually thereafter.

Side effects from statins are often, but not always, class specific. Therefore, side effects from one statin should not discourage a trial with a different statin. Fluvastatin, pravstatin, and atorvastatin seem to have the lowest rates of muscle-related side effects and should be tried first in patients with muscle-related complaints. All episodes of rhabdomyolysis in patients taking simvastatin have occurred with those on the 80 mg per day dosage. No episodes have occurred at lower doses, so simvastatin should rarely be used at the 80 mg dose [7]. If further LDL lowering is required beyond what 40 to 60 mg simvastatin provides, it is safer to switch to combination therapy or another potent statin such as atorvastatin or rosuvastatin.

Prior concerns about statins causing cancer have been alleviated by several meta-analyses of randomized trials of statin therapy that showed no increase in fatal or nonfatal cancers [8,9]. These same meta-analyses also did not show a reduction in cancer. No statins are safe to use during pregnancy.

Usage

Statins are primarily used to lower LDL cholesterol and should be the drugs of first choice for lowering LDL cholesterol because of the tremendous evidence base supporting their use (see Chapter 1). They have a small beneficial effect on raising HDL and lowering TG as well. These effects are most pronounced with rosuvastatin and atorvastatin, respectively.

Pravastatin is the only statin with dual pathways of elimination through the liver and kidney. Pravastatin does not affect CYP450 metabolism and therefore has less interaction with other medications and is preferred when patients are on multiple other medications. Statins should be added if the LDL goal is not reached after 3 months of therapeutic lifestyle changes (TLC) in patients at low or medium risk for coronary artery disease. They should be started simultaneously with TLC in patients at high or very high risk of coronary disease: this includes almost all patients with diabetes.

Fish Oil

Fish oil capsules are available over the counter and recently as a highly concentrated prescription medication, Omacor®. The key oils are omega-3 (n-3) polyunsaturated fatty acids (PUFAs), mainly eicosapentaenoic acid (EPA), and docosahexanoic acid (DHA) [10]. The main dietary source of these oils is from fatty fish such as salmon, but small amounts are also found in nuts, flaxseeds, and canola or flaxseed oils.

Dosage and Actions

The most prominent effects of these fatty acids are to inhibit thrombus formation, decrease inflammation, and lower triglycerides. The over-the-counter formulations of fish oil capsules have amounts of PUFAs ranging from 150 to 500 mg per capsule. The prescription form of fish oil, Omacor®, has 900 mg of PUFAs per capsule. The benefits of fish oil consumption increase with higher doses; however, side effects also increase. Most studies have demonstrated beneficial effects at doses of 1500 to 4000 mg of PUFAs per day.

Fish oil at lower doses has many beneficial effects as an antithrombotic agent. To effectively reduce triglycerides, higher doses are required. The FDA-approved dose of Omacor® to treat hypertriglyceridemia is 4000 mg per day. Daily doses of 3 to 12 g PUFAs can decrease TG by 20% to 50% [10]. The effects on LDL and HDL are generally minimal, although LDL may increase slightly as TGs decrease.

Adverse Effects

Fish oil is usually free of serious side effects. Burping, dyspepsia, a fishy aftertaste, and malodorous sweat are all annoying complaints that are experienced by some patients. Large doses of fish oil can increase bleeding time, so caution should be exercised in the prescription of large doses of fish oil to patients taking anticoagulants. LDL levels may increase modestly during therapy of patients with hypertriglyceridemia.

Omacor®, because of a unique manufacturing process, may cause less burping, aftertaste, and malodorous sweating than over-the-counter forms, but it is more costly. Further, patient-oriented evidence is required to buttress this manufacturer claim.

Usage

Fish oil can be used to treat hypertriglyceridemia as monotherapy or in combination with other lipid-lowering agents such as statins or fibrates. They do not interact with statins (such as gemfibrozil) to increase the risk of rhabdomyolysis, which offers an advantage in patients with elevated levels of both LDL and TG.

Some experts use fish oil for its general beneficial cardiovascular risk modification; however, most of the evidence supporting this is from epidemiologic dietary studies of fish and nut consumption versus large studies of supplement consumption. The Diet and Reinfarction Trial studied survivors of a recent myocardial infarction, finding that those who increased their consumption of fatty fish or fish oil capsules had a 29% relative risk reduction in total mortality in just 2 years [11].

Combination Agents

Dyslipidemia can often involve a lipid profile that has multiple abnormal lipid subfractions. Although statins work well for helping patients reach their individualized LDL targets, they are not as potent at increasing HDL or lowering TG. Some patients require additional agents to reach goal. Generally, compliance is enhanced by combining two agents into a single capsule or tablet.

For example, a combination of a statin and ezetimibe is more effective at LDL lowering than doubling the dosage of the statin and costs less. This approach also has a lower rate of side effects and requires that a patient only add one tablet to their daily pharmacologic regimen. Often, patients with preexisting coronary disease, hypertension, or diabetes are already on several medications. The advantage for compliance and psychological well-being when a physician is able to add only one tablet with dual antilipidemic effects is significant.

Dosage and Actions

Combination drugs currently include ezetimibe + simvastatin (Vytorin®), and niacin + lovastatin (Advicor®). An agent that combines atorvastatin + amlodipine (Caduet® for blood pressure and angina control) also exists. In development are agents that combine atorvastatin with a cholesterol ester transferase protein inhibitor (CETP inhibitor). CETP inhibitors are a new class of agent that can elevate HDL. At present, there is no CETP inhibitor available for use, and trial data are mixed. Although these agents seem to elevate HDL significantly, they have also led to an increase in mortality in some trials. Their eventual utility is unclear at this time.

Vytorin® is available in combinations of 10 mg ezetimibe + 10 mg or 20 mg or 40 mg or 80 mg simvastatin, respectively. It is dosed once per day and can lower LDL by as much as 60% [12].

Advicor® is available in combinations of 20 mg lovastatin and 500 mg niacin or 20 mg lovastatin with 1000 mg niacin. It can be dosed once or twice per day and reduces LDL cholesterol by as much as 45%, reduces TG by 42%, and raises HDL cholesterol by 41% [2].

Usage

The combination agents are most useful for patients who have not achieved their lipid goals with a high dose of a statin or are unable to tolerate a high dose of a statin. In addition, for patients with abnormalities of LDL, TG, and HDL, a combination agent such as Advicor® is very useful. The combination agents are also less costly than prescribing the individual drugs separately.

Agents Used in Combination

Most of the possible combinations of the six classes of agents have been studied in clinical trials. The exception is that ezetimibe has not yet been studied in combination with a fibrate or niacin. Additionally, prescription fish oil (Omacor®) has not been formally studied in combination with other agents. These trials have primarily been designed to test the safety and lipid-lowering efficacy of the combinations as opposed to clinical outcomes. Recently, some of these trials have begun to investigate carotid medial intima thickness regression and other clinical endpoints. Given that most patients are tried on statin agents, most of the research has focused on these regimens. The use of combinations that do not include a statin are limited to patients who cannot tolerate statins.

Statin Combinations

Statins and resins lead to complementary lowering of LDL greater than seen with either agent used alone. Typically, this is in the range of 10% to 20% above that of the statin used alone. Side effects neither increased nor decreased from that seen when the agents were used alone [13].

Statins and fibrates are less potent at reducing LDL than the combination of statins and resins. However, they provide much more effective reduction of TG and elevation of HDL. This combination increases the risk of hepatic transaminase elevation, but this has not led to significant increases in clinical hepatitis. The risk for myositis is also increased, but this increased risk is *primarily when combining gemfibrozil with a statin*. The risk is not significantly increased when combining fenofibrate with a statin [14,15].

Statins and niacin can also be combined. This combination provides even greater elevation in HDL than the combination of a statin with a fibrate. LDL reduction is similar to the combination of a statin with a resin. TG reduction is slightly less than the combination of a statin and a fibrate. Side effects are similar to the agents given separately.

Resins Plus Fibrates

This combination provides better reduction of LDL and TG than the agents used alone. It is less reliable at increasing HDL than a fibrate used alone. There is no increase in side effects with this combination compared with using the agents separately.

Resins Plus Niacin

This combination provides good reduction of both LDL and TG. In contrast to the combination of resins and fibrates, this combination reliably increases HDL as well. There is no increase in side effects from the agents used separately.

Fibrates Plus Niacin

The combination of fibrates plus niacin appears to be safe and effective at lowering LDL and TG and increasing HDL. There is an increase in hepatic enzyme elevation, but not in clinical hepatitis. However, the number of studies of this combination therapy is limited [16].

Combinations of More Than Two Agents

Only a few trials have investigated the utility of combining three or more agents in patients with abnormalities of multiple lipid subfractions. The combinations of a statin plus a resin and a fibrate have been studied as well as the combination of a statin plus a resin and niacin. These trials have shown remarkable improvements in LDL, TG, and HDL, with no significant increase in side effects. As with dual therapy, it is more likely that transaminases will increase with statin–fibrate or statin–niacin combinations, but this increase in transaminases has not correlated with an increase in clinical hepatitis [17].

Drug Interactions, Tolerability, and Severe Side Effects

The goal of this section is to describe general medication class characteristics of agents with regard to safety and tolerability while simultaneously including specific clinically relevant characteristics of individual agents (Tables 6.6, 6.7). The focus is on common side effects and potentially severe reactions associated with agents to treat hyperlipidemia, with an emphasis on myopathy, rhabdomyolysis, and hepatic injury.

Myalgias are a common everyday event for many people and do not necessarily reflect a severe side effect related to therapy. The National Institute of Neurologic Disorders and Stroke (NINDS) has developed useful definitions for understanding types of muscle injury or diseases, termed myopathies (Table 6.8).

The second issue is to define what laboratory values are clinically useful in the evaluation of a possible drug-triggered myopathy. The clinical advisory panel of the American College of Cardiology, the American Heart Association, and the National Heart, Lung and Blood Institute (ACC/AHA/NHLBI) noted that some asymptomatic patients will have moderate [i.e., between 3 and 10 times the upper limit of normal (ULN)] creatinine kinase (CK) elevations at baseline or during treatment. Such patients can usually be treated without harm. However, careful monitoring of symptoms and more frequent CK measurements are indicated. Further, if a physician chooses to obtain CK values in asymptomatic patients, particularly those on combination therapy, and CKs are elevated to more than 10 times the ULN, strong consideration should be given to stopping therapy. Following discontinuation, wait for symptoms to resolve and CK levels to return to normal before reinitiating therapy with a drug and use a lower dose of drug(s) if possible [18].

Elevated hepatic transaminases related to statin (and likely fibrate use) occur in approximately 0.5% to 2.0% of patients on these agents and appear to be dose dependent. Progression to liver failure is exceedingly rare. Regression typically occurs with dose reduction or discontinuation of the agent. It is also important to

Table 6.6 Drug interactions

Medication	Doses for 30%–40% LDL reduction	Metabolism	Drug-comorbidity with diseases	Drug comorbidity with meds	Drug–drug interactions	Drug–other lipid agents
Statins						
Atorvastatin (Lipitor®)	10 mg/day	CYP3A4 Lipophilic Active metabolites	Liver disease No dosage change in chronic kidney disease (CKD) Less than 1% chance of transient proteinuria Pregnancy category: X	Monitor prothrombin (PT) times when receiving Warfarin Verapamil	Azole antifungals HIV protease inhibitors Macrolides Cyclosporin Digoxin	Colestipol lowers plasma concentration by 25 % Fibrates: increased risk of myopathy
Fluvastatin (Lescol®)	40–80 mg/day	CYP2C9 Lipophilic Inactive metabolites	Liver disease No reported fatal rhabdomyolysis events Greater than 40 mg dosing not evaluated with CKD Pregnancy category: X	Monitor PT times when receiving Warfarin Glyburide Digoxin	Diclofenac Ticlopidine Phenytoin H$_2$-antagonist Omeprazole	Cholestyramine decreases fluvastatin if given less than 4 h Less than 1% reported muscle symptoms when used with fibrates. Possibly safest agent for use with fibrates Fibrates: increased risk of myopathy
Lovastatin (Memacor®)	40 mg/day	CYP3A4 Lipophilic Active metabolites	Liver disease 25%–50% reduction in dose with CKD Pregnancy category: X	Monitor PT when receiving Warfarin Verapamil Digoxin	Azole antifungals HIV protease inhibitors Macrolides	
Pravastatin (Pravachol®)	40 mg/day	Sulfation Not lipophilic Moderate protein binding Inactive metabolites	Liver disease Monitor patients with CKD Less than 1% chance of transient proteinuria Pregnancy category: X	Monitor PT when receiving Warfarin Digoxin	Less CYP drug–drug interaction Cyclosporin	Fibrates: Gemfibrozil use not recommended.

Table 6.6 (continued)

Medication	Doses for 30%–40% LDL reduction	Metabolism	Drug-comorbidity with diseases	Drug comorbidity with meds	Drug–drug interactions	Drug–other lipid agents
Rosuvastatin (Crestor®)	5–10 mg/day 80 mg dose withdrawn Do not start at 40 mg dose	Minimal CYP2C9, 2C19 Not lipophilic Minor active metabolites	Liver disease 25%–50% reduction in dose Do not exceed 10 mg/day in kidney disease patients. Pregnancy category: X	Monitor PT when receiving Warfarin Digoxin	Less CYP interaction Diclofenac Ticlopidine Cyclosporin	Fibrates: increased risk of myopathy
Simvastatin (Zocor®)	5–80 mg dose Doses more than 40 mg with greater side effects	CYP3A4	Liver disease Rhabdomyolysis risk as monotherapy almost exclusively with 80 mg dose	Monitor PT when receiving Warfarin Digoxin	Cyclosporin macrolides Azole antifungals	Fibrates: increased risk of myopathy. Keep dose below 20 mg/day with gemfibrozil
Bile acid sequestrants (resins)						
Cholestyramine (Questran®)	4–24 g/day (1–6 packets or scoops)	Not absorbed	Constipation Patients with bowel obstruction Not studied with elevated TG levels (greater than 300 mg/dl) Not indicated for familial abetalipoproteinemia or genetic hypobeta-lipoproteinemia Pregnancy category C	Potential binding Glipizide Thiazide diuretics Propranolol	Bioavailability effect on: Valproic acid Phenobarbitol Penicillin G Estrogens Progerstins Phenylbutazone	Additive effects demonstrated with the following statins: Pravastatin Fluvastatin Lovastatin Demonstrated benefit with niacin 750 mg/day Demonstrated benefit with the following fibrates: • Gemfibrozil • Bezafibrate

Table 6.6 (continued)

Medication	Doses for 30%–40% LDL reduction	Metabolism	Drug-comorbidity with diseases	Drug comorbidity with meds	Drug–drug interactions	Drug–other lipid agents
Colestipol (Colestid®)	Powder: 5–30 g/day (1–6 packets) Tablet: 2–16 g/day (2–16 tablets)	Not absorbed	Constipation Patients with bowel obstruction Not studied with elevated TG levels (greater than 300 mg/dl) Not indicated for familial abetalipoproteinemia or genetic hypobetalipoproteinemia Pregnancy category C	Thiazide diuretics Propranolol Furosemide Digoxin Diltiazem	Bioavailability effect on: Tetracycline Penicillin G Diclofenac	Additive effects demonstrated with the following statins: • Lovastatin • Simvastatin Demonstrated benefit with niacin 3–12 g/day Demonstrated benefit with Fenofibrate Reduces levels of Ezetimibe
Colesevelam (Welchol®)	3.8–4.5 g/day (6–7 tablets)	Not absorbed	Patients with bowel obstruction Not studied with elevated TG levels (greater than 300 mg/dl) Not indicated for familial abetalipoproteine-mia or genetic hypo-betalipoproteinemia Pregnancy category B	Verapamil		Additive effects demonstrated with the following statins: • Lovastatin • Simvastatin • Atorvastatin Demonstrated added benefit with Fenofibrate Demonstrated benefit with Ezetimibe
Nicotinic acid (niacin) Immediate-release nicotinic acid	1.5–30 g/day	Primary pathway: Conjugative forming nicotinuric acid (flushing) Secondary pathway: Oxidation-reduction yielding nicoti-namide/pyrimidines (hepatotoxicity)	Hepatotoxicity Caution use in patients with diabetes (association with hyperglycemia and insulin resistance), anticoagulants, alcohol use, gout Monitor for myopathy Pregnancy category C		Cyclosporine	Benefits demonstrated with cholestyramine, colestipol, and statins Caution with statins and fibrates

Table 6.6 (continued)

Medication	Doses for 30%–40% LDL reduction	Metabolism	Drug–comorbidity with diseases	Drug comorbidity with meds	Drug–drug interactions	Drug–other lipid agents
Extended-release nicotinic acid (Niaspan®) 1-2	1–2 g/day	Balanced metabolism between the two pathways	Lower incidence of hepatotoxicity compared to IR and SR preparations Caution use in patients with diabetes (association with hyperglycemia and insulin resistance), anticoagulants, alcohol use, gout Monitor for myopathy Pregnancy category C		Cyclosporine	Benefits demonstrated with cholestyramine, colestipol, and statins Caution with statins and fibrates
Long-acting nicotinic acid	1–2 g/day	Primary pathway: Oxidation-reduction pathway (high affinity-low capacity) yielding nicotinamide and pyrimidines (hepatotoxicity)	Hepatotoxicity (52% incidence in one study, 67% withdrew) Caution use in patients with diabetes (association with hyperglycemia and insulin resistance), anticoagulants, alcohol use, gout Monitor for myopathy Pregnancy category C		Cyclosporine	Benefits demonstrated with cholestyramine, colestipol, and statins Caution with statins and fibrates

Table 6.6 (continued)

Medication	Doses for 30%–40% LDL reduction	Metabolism	Drug-comorbidity with diseases	Drug comorbidity with meds	Drug–drug interactions	Drug–other lipid agents
Fibrates						
Gemfibrozil (Lopid®)	600 mg bid	Extensive liver metabolism Oxidation via CYP450 2C8 Highly protein bound Renal excretion	Do not use in preexisting gallbladder disease Caution with hepatic dysfunction Caution with severe renal impairment Pregnancy category C	Glyburide (hypoglycemia) Pioglitazone (Increase in pioglitazone and hypoglycemia) Rosiglitazone (same) Warfarin (including bleeding)	Extreme caution with statins Colestipol (decreased gemfibrozil effectiveness) Ezetimibe (increased Ezetimide levels, risk of gallstones)	Demonstrated benefit with cholestyramine
Fenofibrate	Lipofen: 50–150 mg qd Tricor: 48–145 mg qd Triglide: 160 mg Lofibra-(micronized): 200 mg qd	Glucuronidation Little CYP450 Renal excretion Highly protein bound	Do not use in preexisting gallbladder disease Caution with hepatic disease Caution with severe CKD May cause homocysteinemia Pregnancy category C	Warfarin	One-third dose with geriatric patients and renal disease Caution with statins Cholestyramine decreases fenofibrat Caution with cyclosporine (renal) Administer 1 h before or 6 h after colesevelam and colestipol With ezetimibe, may increase gallstones	Demonstrated added benefit with colestipol and colesevelam Lower rhabdo rate with statins compared to other fibrates (0.58 per million prescriptions vs. 8.6 per million prescriptions of gemfibrozil)

Table 6.6 (continued)

Medication	Doses for 30%–40% LDL reduction	Metabolism	Drug-comorbidity with diseases	Drug comorbidity with meds	Drug–drug interactions	Drug–other lipid agents
Clofibrate (Atromid®)	1000 mg bid	Glucuronidation Renal excretion	Caution with renal disease: q 18 h dosing with moderate renal impairment q 24–48 h with renal failure Caution with liver failure	Glyburide (hypoglycemia) Insulins (hypoglycemia) Furosemide (myalgia, increased LAE and diuretic effects)	Chlorpropamide (hypoglycemia) Fosphenytoin and phenytoin (elevated phenytoin levels)	Ezetimide (gallstones) Statins (myopathy) Tolazemide (hypoglycemia) Tolbutamide (hypoglycemia) Warfarin (increased bleeding)
Cholesterol absorption inhibitors						
Ezetimibe (Zetia®)	10 mg	Inhibit cholesterol absorption Glucuronidation No evident effect on drug metabolism enzymes	Possibly age-related (over 75 years) side effect: increased transaminase levels; increased discontinuation over age 75 (12% vs. 3% less than 75 years old)	Not evident at this time	Cholestyramine reduces plasma concentration of ezetimibe	Demonstrated benefit with colesevelam Likely additive effects with statins

Source: Data from Pasternak RC, Smith SC, Bairey-Merz CN, Grundy SM, Cleeman JI, Lenfant C. ACC/AHA/NHLBI clinical advisory on the use and safety of statins. J Am Coll Cardiol 2002:40(3):568–573; Jones PH, Davidson MH. Reporting rate of rhabdomyolysis with fenofibrate + statin versus gemfibrozil + any statin. Am J Cardiol 2005:95:120–122; Insull W. Clinical utility of bile acid sequestrants in the treatment of dyslipidemia: a scientific review. South Med J 2006;99(3):257–272; Miller M. Niacin as a component of combination therapy for dyslipidemia. Mayo Clin Proc 2003;78:735–742; MICROMEDEX (2006). DRUGDEX Evaluations: Ezetimibe.

Table 6.7 Drug tolerability and potentially severe side effects

Medication	Tolerability and common minor side effects	Potentially severe side effects
Statins	Generally well tolerated Possibly increased discontinuation at higher doses Dose dependent elevations in hepatic transaminases (0.5%–2.0%) Myalgias ~5% Generally less than 5% discontinuation rates	Severe myopathy: approximately 1/1000 Fatal rhabdomyolysis; 1 death/million prescriptions Liver failure: rare
Bile acid sequestrants (resins)	Constipation and GI side effects	Potential binding of coadministered medication
Nicotinic acid (niacin)	Flushing Nausea, vomiting, diarrhea Hyperglycemia Acanthosis nigricans Hyperuricemia and gout	Hepatotoxicity Activation of peptic ulcer disease
Fibric acid (fibrates)	Generally well tolerated Rash (about 8%) GI: diarrhea, flatulence, nausea/vomiting (less than 10%) Myalgias Rhinitis	Pancreatitis (rare) Hepatotoxicity (rare) Rhabdomyolysis (rare)
Cholesterol absorption inhibitor	Current side effect profile comparable to placebo	Avoid in moderate-severe hepatic impairment

Source: Data from Pasternak RC, Smith SC, Bairey-Merz CN, Grundy SM, Cleeman JI, Lenfant C. ACC/AHA/NHLBI clinical advisory on the use and safety of statins. J Am Coll Cardiol 2002;40(3):568–573; CTT Collaborators. Efficacy and safety of cholesterol-lowering treatment: prospective meta-analysis of data from 90056 participants in 14 randomised trials of statins. Lancet 2005;366:1267–1278; Jacobson T. Overcoming "ageism" bias in the treatment of hyper-cholesterolemia: a review of safety issues with statins in the elderly. Drug Saf 2006;29(5): 421–448; Jones PH, Davidson MH. Reporting rate of rhabdomyolysis with fenofibrate + statin versus gemfibrozil + any statin. Am J Cardiol 2005;95:120–122; Insull W. Clinical utility of bile acid sequestrants in the treatment of dyslipidemia: a scientific review. South Med J 2006;99(3):257–272; Miller M. Niacin as a component of combination therapy for dyslipidemia. Mayo Clin Proc 2003;78:735–742; MICROMEDEX (2006). DRUGDEX Evaluations: Ezetimibe; Bruckert E, Giral P, Tellier P. Perspectives in cholesterol-lowering therapy. The role of Ezetimibe, a new selective inhibitor of intestinal cholesterol absorption. Circulation 2003;107:3124–3128.

consider other medications, alcohol intake, or foods the patient may be consuming that might result in transaminase abnormalities.

Medications and conditions associated with an increased risk for statin-related myopathy are listed in Table 6.9. This list should not be considered as absolute contraindications for these medications that have profound preventive and therapeutic benefit; this list should simply alert the clinician for consideration of treatment benefits, effectiveness, and side effects. Table 6.10 outlines a clinical approach to monitoring statin therapy and addressing side effects.

Table 6.8 Myopathy definitions

Myalgia: Muscle ache or weakness without creatinine kinase (CK) elevation
Myositis: Muscle symptoms with increased CK levels
Rhabdomyolysis: Muscle symptoms with marked CK elevations [typically substantially greater than 10 times the upper limit of normal (ULN) and with creatinine elevation (usually with brown urine and urinary myoglobin)]

Source: Data from Pasternak RC, Grundy SM, Smith SC, et al. ACC/AHA/NHLBI clinical advisory on the safety and use of statins. J Am Coll Cardiol 2002;40:568–573.

Table 6.9 Risk factors for statin-associated myopathy

Advanced age (greater than 80 years), especially women
Small frame, sarcopenia, nutritional and functional compromise (frailty)
Multisystem diseases and associated polypharmacy
Perioperative or perihospitalization periods
The following medications/agents:

- Fibrates (especilly gemfibrozil)
- Cyclosporine
- Azole antifungals
- Itraconazole and ketoconazol
- Macrolide antibiotics
- HIV protease inhibitors
- Nefazodone
- Verapamil
- Amiodarone

Source: From Pasternak RC, Smith SC, Bairey-Merz CN, Grundy SM, Cleeman JI, Lenfant C. ACC/AHA/NHLBI clinical advisory on the use and safety of statins. J Am Coll Cardiol 2002; 40(3):568–573.

Table 6.10 A clinical approach to monitoring and follow-up of therapy with statins

Indication for statin?	Perform risk assessment
Baseline labs:	Lipids, complete metabolic profile, CK
Start therapy.	
Check liver functions at 6 weeks:	Lipids and liver functions at 12 weeks
Meeting goals?	Adjust therapy to meet goals by dose increase or adding agent
Muscle symptoms?	Check CK, TSH, and evaluate other possible causes of symptoms
If CK less than three times ULN:	Continue to monitor, advise moderation in physical activity as applicable
CK 3–10 times ULN?	Continue to monitor weekly until spontaneous resolution, or discontinue if worsens
CK greater than 10 times normal?	Consider: Discontinuation or reduction in therapy, reevaluate need for therapy, possible interactions, alternate agents, or resumption of statin therapy.
If liver functions less than 3 times normal:	Continue therapy
If liver functions increased:	Recheck every 6 weeks until stabilized

ULN, upper limit of normal.

Statins

Safety

The primary safety concern for the statins is for the development of muscle injury syndromes within the continuum of myalgias, cramps, myolysis, myositis, and myopathy. Hepatic injury manifested by elevations in transaminases is also associated with these agents. Rash, headaches, and gastrointestinal disturbances can occur with these agents, but are usually self-limited.

Muscle injury associated with statins is a class effect and possibly caused by reduced function of the mitochondrial energy-producing apparatus in skeletal muscle. Myalgia happens in 1% to 5% of patients receiving statins and typically decreases with dose reduction or discontinuation. Myositis is associated with muscle weakness and greater than 10-fold elevation in CK. There is an approximate 1:1000 chance of developing myositis (at greater than 10-fold elevation in CK) with lovastatin, simvastatin, and pravastatin [18]. Resultant rhabdomyolysis from randomized controlled trials suggests a 0.023% risk of rhabdomyolysis with statins versus 0.015% risk with placebo, with a small and insignificant increased risk of rhabdomyolysis over 5 years [19]. In other terms, rates of mortality related to rhabdomyolysis are less than 1 per million prescriptions [20].

Polypharmacy is very common in the elderly, and medications with cytochrome P metabolism must be specially monitored. Fibric acid derivatives likely increase the systemic exposure to statins and must be especially watched for myopathy. The ACC/AHA/NHBLI advisory cites one study of combined statin and fibrate (primarily gemfibrozil) in which 1% of patients developed CK elevations greater than three times normal without muscle symptoms, and 1% withdrew from therapy for reasons of muscle discomfort, with no cases of rhabdomyolysis in the reported studies. Fenofibrate is associated with lower risk as compared to gemfibrozil, which makes it the agent of choice when combining a statin and a fibrate [21].

Hepatic toxicity is thought to be strongly associated with advancing age or increasing statin dose. Checking liver-associated enzymes before therapy and after therapy initiation or dose changes is therefore recommended. By definition, drug-associated hepatocellular injury is not present unless ALT and AST levels increase to more than three times the upper limit of normal and bilirubin levels to more than two times the upper limit of normal over a 12-month period. The natural history of maintenance of statin therapy with persistent transaminase elevations is not known, but typically levels normalize with dose decrease or discontinuation.

Tolerability

Trials of individual statins demonstrate discontinuation rates similar to placebo, although there are potentially significant differences in discontinuation rates with high dose therapy of some statins. For this reason, combination therapy of a statin (at moderate dose) plus another agent may be more beneficial in treating the patient not meeting cholesterol goals. Maximal monotherapy with a statin may only increase risk of side effects.

Bile Acid Sequestrants

Safety

Few systemic side effects are noted with these agents. The potential drug-binding properties of these agents result in possible ineffectiveness of other agents to treat comorbid conditions.

Tolerability

Tolerability of cholestyramine is limited by significant gastrointestinal symptoms to include flatulence and constipation, which appears to be dose dependent. Palatability and complicated dosing schedules to avoid interactions with other medications result in discontinuation rates of 40% to 60%. Eleven percent of colesevelam patients report constipation and dyspepsia [22].

Fibrates

Safety

Concerns for fibrate toxicity surround the rare incidence of myopathy during monotherapy and rhabdomyolysis when fibrates are used in combination with statins. Hepatotoxicity and pancreatitis are also rare occurrences with fibrates. Fenofibrate appears to have a much lower rate of occurrence of rhabdomyolysis than gemfibrozil.

Tolerability

Fibrates are generally well tolerated. Gastrointestinal (GI) upset is reported in less than 10% of patients. Rash may occur with fibrate therapy in approximately 8% of patients.

Niacin

Safety

The primary safety concern of the niacin derivatives is hepatotoxicity, with one study demonstrating 67% withdrawal from therapy with the *long-acting* preparations as a consequence of elevated liver enzymes. Dose should be retitrated if switching brands or changing from immediate- to sustained-release niacin.

Extended-release niacin demonstrated only a 5% elevation of liver-associated enzymes and a reduced incidence of flushing [23]. Caution should be exercised in those patients with a history of gout and peptic ulcer disease. Lower risk of myopathy is apparent with statin + nicotinic acid (except extended-release preparations) than with gemfibrozil + statin combinations.

Tolerability

Facial and truncal flushing is common and can result in discontinuation of therapy in 25% of patients [23]. Aspirin (325 mg) or other nonsteroidal antiinflammatory medications taken 30 to 60 min before the first dose of niacin reduced this event, as well as slow upward titration of the dosage. Sustained-release preparations decrease flushing but have a much greater risk of hepatotoxicity.

Absorption Inhibitors

Safety

There is currently no evidence of interaction with drug metabolism enzymes and interaction potential seems to be low; this includes interactions with warfarin, glipizide, digoxin, oral contraceptives, and statins. The medication is not recommended in those with moderate or greater hepatic impairment. No dose changes appear to be necessary for renal impairment when used as monotherapy.

Tolerability

Initial and postmarketing studies suggest excellent tolerability when compared to placebo [24,25].

Drug–Food Side Effects

Grapefruit Juice and Hyperlipidemia Therapy

Health-conscious individuals may be consuming a variety of foods to reduce cholesterol, reduce weight, or lower blood pressure. One possible side effect of this behavior change is that an individual may potentially encounter drug–food side effects. A common concern for hyperlipidemia therapy is the suppressive action that grapefruit and grapefruit juice exerts on intestinal CYP3A4, a common enzyme used by many drugs in metabolism. This suppression may result in higher drug levels of atorvastatin, lovastatin, and simvastatin. The Center for Food and Drug Interaction developed by the University of Florida is a great resource for patients and providers to explore for useful information on this phenomenon (www.druginteractioncenter.com).

Clinician actions can include the following recommendations to patients:

- Switching to orange juice
- Switching to ezetimibe, colesevelam, or niacin
- Lowering the dose of the current statin and reducing grapefruit ingestion to an occasional small glass of grapefruit juice or a half-grapefruit

Drugs of the Future

Despite the choices available for the pharmacologic treatment of dyslipidemia, many patients have lipid subfractions that are resistant to reduction to optimum levels. Three common issues include difficulty in reducing LDL to less than 70 mg/dl, reducing TG to less than 150 mg/dl, and raising HDL to greater than 40 mg/dl. Research has focused on the development of new agents to ameliorate these problems.

Additionally, many patients with metabolic syndrome commonly have dyslipidemia, obesity, glucose intolerance, and hypertension, which has led to research in agents that can simultaneously treat all these problems.

Greater LDL Reduction

Research continues on a new class of statins termed "super-statins." At present, the closest to FDA approval is pitavastatin [26]. This agent is already available in Japan. It has greater LDL-lowering potential than rosuvastatin and a greater effect on raising HDL and TG. It also has a different pathway of metabolism, which should lead to fewer drug–drug interactions than other statins, similar to the rate seen with pravastatin. Other agents combining statins and ezetimibe or statins and niacin are also in development. Each of these should increase the ability to reduce LDL further.

Greater HDL Elevation

Raising HDL is difficult with the agents currently available. Inhibition of cholesterol ester transferase protein (CETP) is a method to directly increase HDL. Torcetrapib is a CETP inhibitor that can raise HDL from 40% to 100% [27]. Although the ability of torcetrapib to increase HDL safely seems assured, the only clinical outcome study done to prove that the HDL produced is biologically active at reducing ASCVD was terminated as a result of unexpected increase in mortality in the CETP-treated group.

HDL expresses apolipoprotein A-1 on its surface. It is known that levels of apolipoprotein A-1 are inversely related to coronary events. Drugs that increase the expression and levels of apolipoprotein A-1 are also in development. Currently, ETC-216 (recombinant apolipoprotein milano) has been shown to raise HDL and apolipoprotein A-1 and cause a regression in atherosclerosis [28].

Many of the drugs that raise HDL do so through effects on reverse cholesterol transport. In development are a variety of pharmacologic substances that inhibit or catalyze enzymes along this reverse cholesterol pathway; these include lecithin cholesterol acyltransferase (LCAT) promoters, adenosine triphosphate-binding cassette protein A1 (ABCA1) promoters, scavenger receptor class-B1 protein inhibitors (SR-B1), lipoprotein lipase promoters, and hepatic lipase inhibitors. Promoting or inhibiting each of these proteins leads to an increase in HDL levels [29].

Research also continues on formulations of niacin that cause fewer side effects. Niacin is remarkably effective at increasing HDL. It has been the side effects of high niacin doses that have limited its usefulness. Extended-release formulations, innovative capsule layering technology, and less frequent dosing are all approaches that may improve the utility of niacin.

Agents with Multiple Actions

Fibrates act on perioxisome proliferators antagonist receptor-alpha (PPAR-α) to raise HDL and lower TG. Thiazolidinedione agents affect perioxisome proliferators antagonist receptor-gamma (PPAR-γ) and can reduce blood sugar, insulin resistance, weight, and blood pressure. Research on agents that affect PPARs more selectively is ongoing. Muraglitazaar is an agent that is an agonist for both PPAR-α and PPAR-γ. It helps reduce both glucose and TG. However, it unpredictably increased cardiovascular events in patients with type 2 diabetes, leading to a suspension of its use while this was further investigated [30]. Currently, research continues on single and dual PPAR agonists because these agents have the promise of multiple risk factor reduction through the use of a single agent.

Cannabinoid-1 Receptor Antagonists

Cannabinoid receptors modulate appetite suppression directly and weight, glucose levels, and lipids indirectly, but potently in vitro. Several trials have been undertaken to see if the cannabinoid receptor antagonist rimonabant can affect all these cardiovascular risk parameters in patients [31].

The Rimonabant in Obesity Trials (RIO trials) have studied this agent. RIO-LIPID specifically looked at the effects of rimonabant on lipids; it reduced TG by 13%, increased HDL by 19%, but it also increased LDL by 7%. There was no change in glucose noted [31]. This trial has somewhat tempered enthusiasm for the use of this agent for the specific treatment of dyslipidemia, yet the promise of this class of agents remains because of their novel mechanism of action.

Immunosuppression to Reduce Atherosclerosis

A revolutionary approach to the reduction of atherosclerosis is to induce tolerance to elevated levels of lipids in the serum. Trials have been undertaken in animal models to induce immune suppression and tolerance to high levels of oxidized LDL, which is the most potent inducer of systemic atherosclerosis [32]. These early animal trials are encouraging and point toward a completely different approach to the prevention of ASCVD that targets the actual process of atherosclerosis versus the reduction of the raw materials—namely lipids—that fuel this process. Success in this arena is likely still decades away.

References

1. Choice of lipid regulating drugs. Med Lett 2001;43:43–48.
2. Three new drugs for hyperlipidemia. Med Lett 2003;45:17–19.
3. McKenney JM, Proctor JD, Harris S, et al. A comparison of the efficacy and toxic effects of sustained release vs. immediate release niacin in hypercholesterolemic patients. JAMA 1994;271:672–677.
4. Staffa JA, Cahng J, Green L. Cerivistatin and reports of fatal rhabdomyolysis. N Engl J Med 2002;346:539–540.
5. Thompson PD, Clarkson P, Karas RH. Statin-associated myopathy. JAMA 2003;289: 1681–1690.
6. Pasternak RC, Smith SC, Bairey-Merz CN, Grundy SM, Cleeman JI, Lenfant C. ACC/AHA/NHLBI clinical advisory on the safety and use of statins. J Am Coll Cardiol 2002;40:568–573.
7. Lemos JA, Blazing MA, Wiviott SD, et al. Early intensive vs. a delayed conservative simvastatin strategy in patients with acute coronary syndromes: phase Z of the A to Z trial. N Engl J Med 2004;292:1307–1316.
8. Bjerre LM, LeLorier J. Do statins cause cancer? Am J Med 2001;110:716–723.
9. Anonymous. Efficacy and safety of cholesterol lowering treatment: prospective meta-analysis of data from 90,056 participants in 14 randomized trials of statins. Lancet 2005;366: 1267–1277.
10. Fish oil supplements. Med Lett 2006;48:59–60.
11. Burr ML, Fehily AM, Gilbert JF, et al. Effects of changes in fat, fish and fibre intakes on death and myocardial reinfarction: Diet and Reinfarction Trial (DART). Lancet 1989;2:757–761.
12. Vytorin. Med Lett 2004;46:73–74.
13. Kweiterovich PO. Review of lipid modifying drugs used alone or in combination. Adv Stud Med 2005;5:475–491.
14. Telford M. Clinical pharmacokinetics of fenofibrate. Curr Med Res Opin 2003;19:139–140.
15. Vega GL, Ma PT, Cater NB, et al. Effects of adding fenofibrate to simvastatin in patients with combined hyperlipidemia and metabolic syndrome. Am J Cardiol 2003;91:956–960.
16. Spencer GA, Wirebaugh S, Whitney EJ. Effect of a combination of gemfibrozil and niacin on lipid levels. J Clin Pharmacol 1996;36:696–700.
17. Brown BG, Bardsley J, Poulin D, et al. Moderate dose three-drug therapy with niacin, lovastatin and colestipol to reduce low density lipoprotein cholesterol <less than>100 mg/dL in patients. Am J Cardiol 1997;80:111–115.
18. Pasternak RC, Smith SC, Bairey-Merz CN, Grundy SM, Cleeman JI, Lenfant C. 2002 ACC/AHA/NHLBI clinical advisory on the use and safety of statins. J Am Coll Cardiol 2002; 40(3):568–573.
19. CTT Collaborators. Efficacy and safety of cholesterol-lowering treatment: prospective meta-analysis of data from 90056 participants in 14 randomised trials of statins. Lancet. 2005;366:1267–1278.
20. Jacobson, T. Overcoming "ageism" bias in the treatment of hypercholesterolemia: a review of safety issues with statins in the elderly. Drug Saf 2006; 29(5):421–448.

21. Jones PH, Davidson MH. Reporting rate of rhabdomyolysis with fenofibrate + statin versus gemfibrozil + any statin. Am J Cardiol 2005; 95:120–122.
22. Insull W. Clinical utility of bile acid sequestrants in the treatment of dyslipidemia: a scientific review. South Med J 2006; 99(3):257–272.
23. Miller M. Niacin as a component of combination therapy for dyslipidemia. Mayo Clin Proc 2003; 78:735–742.
24. MICROMEDEX (2006). DRUGDEX Evaluations: Ezetimibe.
25. Bruckert E, Giral P, Tellier P. Perspectives in cholesterol-lowering therapy. The role of ezetimibe, a new selective inhibitor of intestinal cholesterol absorption. Circulation 2003;107:3124–3128.
26. Saito Y, Yamada N, Teramoto T, et al. A randomized, double blind trial comparing the efficacy and safety of pitavastatin versus pravastatin in patients with primary hypercholesterolemia. Atherosclerosis 2002;162:373–379.
27. Brousseau ME, Schaefer EJ, Wolfe ML, et al. Effects of an inhibitor of cholesterol ester transfer protein on HDL cholesterol. N Engl J Med 2004;350:1505–1515.
28. Nissen SE, Tsunoda T, Tuzcu EM, et al. Effect of recombinant ApoA-1 Milano on coronary atherosclerosis in patients with acute coronary syndromes: a randomized controlled trial. JAMA 2003;290:2292–2300.
29. Rader DJ. Regulation of reverse cholesterol transport and clinical implications. Am J Cardiol 2003;92(4A):42J–49J.
30. Nissen SE, Wolski K, Topol EJ. Effect of muraglitazar on death and major adverse cardiovascular events in patients with type 2 diabetes mellitus. JAMA 2005;294:2581–2586.
31. Gadde KM, Allison DB. Cannabinoid-1 receptor antagonist, Rimonabant, for management of obesity and related risks. Circulation 2006;114:974–984.
32. Goronzy JJ, Weyand CM. Immunosuppression in atherosclerosis: mobilizing the opposition within. Circulation 2006;114:1901–1904.

Suggested Key Readings

Medical Letter on Drugs and Therapeutics; all editions on lipid regulating drugs. Can be accessed at: www.medicalletter.com.
Pasternak RC, Smith SC, Bairey-Merz CN, Grundy SM, Cleeman JI, Lenfant C. ACC/AHA/NHLBI clinical advisory on the safety and use of statins. J Am Coll Cardiol 2002;40:568–573.

Chapter 7
Special Populations

Brian V. Reamy, Brian K. Unwin, and Christopher G. Jarvis

Elderly

This elderly population is a high-risk, problem-prone group that often has multiple comorbidities requiring a comprehensive and caring approach in management to prevent disease and disability. It is also relevant to discuss this population subset because the elderly are the fastest growing demographic subgroup in the U.S. population.

In 2000, 40% of all deaths in Americans over the age of 65 were linked to hyperlipidemia. Coronary artery disease mortality and morbidity are highest among elderly men and women, with more than 80% of the deaths from coronary heart disease (CHD) occurring in individuals over the age of 65 [1]. Reducing the death or resultant disability related to these conditions is of obvious importance and benefit to individual patients and to our nation.

Pharmacologic therapy for hyperlipidemia in elderly patients is expensive for those seniors on limited incomes or with significant drug cost shares. The number of medications and multiple comorbidities common in seniors also complicates hyperlipidemia therapy because of potential interactions between medications.

Healthy People 2010

Before considering medical treatment of hyperlipidemia in older individuals, it is reasonable to consider larger societal healthcare goals for this population. Relevant goals for the treatment of hyperlipidemia from the Healthy People 2010 initiative include the following:

- Fewer than 20% of adults having no leisure-time physical activity
- At least 50% of adults age 65+ eating five or more fruits and vegetables daily

B.V. Reamy
Chair and Associate Professor, Department of Family Medicine, Uniformed Services University of the Health Sciences, Bethesda, MD
e-mail: breamy@usuhs.mil

B.V. Reamy (ed.), *Hyperlipidemia Management for Primary Care*,
DOI: 10.1007/978-0-387-76606-5_7, © Springer Science+Business Media, LLC 2008

- Fewer than 15% of adults experiencing obesity [body mass index (BMI) 30 or more]
- Fewer than 12% of adults currently smoking
- Eighty percent or greater of the adult population having cholesterol checked within 5 years

The 2002 report card on America's seniors for attaining these goals showed that seniors are not getting enough physical activity (32.9%), are eating inadequate amounts of fruits and vegetables (32.4%), and that many are obese (19.5%). Older adults are meeting Healthy People 2010 goals with regards to current smoking (only 10.1% smoked in 2002) and cholesterol checks (85.4% were screened in 2001) [2].

Normal Physiological Aging

Atherosclerotic risk factors are intensified by the aging process. Advanced age itself is an independent risk factor for CHD death. Blood pressure increases with age, as does fat mass, with a corresponding decrease in lean muscle mass. These changes can predispose to the metabolic syndrome and adult-onset diabetes. An additional challenge in the study of atherogenesis in the elderly is to distinguish change caused by normal biological aging ("primary aging") from those changes resulting from lifestyle ("secondary aging") from those factors caused by disease ("tertiary aging"). The context of treatment of geriatric dyslipidemia is to prevent the effects of secondary and tertiary aging.

In general, it is thought that total cholesterol and low density lipoprotein cholesterol (LDL-C) levels in men rise until approximately 40 to 50 years of age, after which there is a slow decline. In women, levels of total cholesterol and LDL-C rise until age 60 to 70 years in the absence of hormone replacement therapy. Data from the National Center of Health Care Statistics from 1999 show a peaking of average total cholesterol for men in the age 45 to 54 cohort at 215 mg/dl and at age 65 to 74 for women with a mean value of 224 mg/dl. High density lipoprotein (HDL) cholesterol generally remains stable throughout an individual's life. Triglyceride levels peak in the mid-forties to mid-fifties in men and in the mid-fifties to mid-sixties in women [3].

Renal Function

Aging results in many structural and functional changes best characterized as a decrease in reserve or resilience. The kidneys are subject to such changes, but, in the absence of significant disease or injury, retain the ability to manage fluid and electrolyte balance into the ninth and tenth decade and beyond. Physiological changes to the kidneys associated with aging include decreases in glomerular filtration rate, renal blood flow, and maximal urinary concentration ability. These changes make the elder patient more susceptible to insult from illness or exposure to toxic agents, to include well-intentioned prescribing of pharmaceuticals [4]. One of the most important geriatric prescribing practices is to always account for decreased renal function and possible drug–drug or drug–disease interactions before initiating or changing medications in an elderly patient.

Liver Function

In general, the gastrointestinal tract retains significant reserve and capacity with aging, with the exception of a notable increase in the frequency of constipation and cholelithiasis. Physiological aging is associated with impaired neuromuscular coordination of the oropharynx, esophageal dysmotility, decreased stomach cyto-protection, decreased exocrine pancreatic function, and altered drug metabolism in the liver.

Generally, typical measurements of hepatic function (liver-associated enzymes) are preserved with aging. The cytochrome P450 system is critical in drug metabo-lism, and in particular the CYP3A subfamily. CYP3A activity is typically reduced in elderly individuals and is particularly important in the metabolism of a number of common agents used in geriatric patients such as calcium channel blockers, immunosuppressants, cholesterol-lowering agents, benzodiazepines, macrolide antibiotics, and nonsedating antihistamines. Thus, the risk of drug interactions and toxicities rise with aging.

The other major significant factor to consider in treatment of hyperlipidemia is to consider the relative loss of lean (muscle) mass, with the relative increase in adipose tissue. With this decline in muscle mass (estimated at 6% per decade between ages 30 and 80), body weight is typically maintained or gained with accu-mulation of adipose tissue, especially with central distribution. This accumulation of adipose tissue places the patient at significant risk for developing frank obesity or metabolic derangements such as hyperlipidemia, adult-onset diabetes, and hyper-tension.

Hypercholesterolemia and the Oldest-Old (Age Greater Than 85 Years)

If the goal of lipid treatment is to prevent premature death, the issue of treating older adults who have exceeded normal life expectancy becomes complicated and contro-versial. As noted later in this chapter, statin therapy has shown protective cardiac benefits in the elderly population with therapy as short as 1 year and probable cere-brovascular benefit with longer therapy (5 years). No prospective lipid treatment trial is known at this time to exist for individuals over the age of 85. Interestingly, two population studies point out that hypercholesterolemia may be protective in this population.

The Weverling-Rijnsburger et al. report in 1997 describes a study of 724 patients with a mean age of 89 followed for 10 years from 1986 to 1996 (Leiden 85-Plus Study). Cholesterol concentration was determined in each individual and was categorized into three groups: less than 5.0 mmol/l (193 mg/dl), 5.0–6.4 mmol/l (247 mg/dl), and 6.5 mmol/l or more (251 mg/dl or more). Of the participants, 89% died in the 10 years of follow-up. After adjusting for age and gender, each 1 mmol/l increase of total cholesterol corresponded to a 15% decrease in mortality. Cardiovascular disease was still the most common cause of death in this study, but it was independent of total serum cholesterol concentration. The lower all-cause mortality in the high cholesterol group was associated with lower mortality risk from cancer and infection. The statistically significant median survival of participants was 2.5 years in the lowest cholesterol category, 3.4 years in the middle category, and 4.3 years in the highest category [5]. The authors of this study and of another supporting population study by Shipley pose that the importance of cholesterol concentration in the oldest-old may be different and *may not reflect* their individual lifetime cholesterol concentration [6]. The authors of the Weverling-Rijnsburger study suggest that LDL cholesterol may have some form of immunomodulatory effect. The authors conclude that a "conclusion about the balance between the benefit and risk of cholesterol-lowering therapy in the oldest has yet to be reached [5]".

Principles of Geriatric Prescribing

Medications to treat hyperlipidemia have demonstrated clear benefit in older adults. However, the decision to prescribe a lipid-lowering agent to an older patient requires significant deliberation by the provider because of the disease and pharmacologic burden carried by older patients. Older Americans make up 13% of the population yet consume 30% of all prescription medications. The majority of older Americans take an average of three to five medications, not counting dietary supplements and over-the-counter (OTC) medications. Patients older than age 80 are commonly hospitalized for adverse drug events.

High-risk older adults include those over the age of 85, those having six or more active medical diagnoses, those having decreased kidney function [creatinine clearance (CrCl) less than 50 ml/min], those having low body weight or body mass index, those taking nine or more active medications, those having previous adverse drug reaction, and those taking more than 12 doses of medication per day [7].

Cultural, psychological, and cost barriers may also impair effective treatment of hyperlipidemia. Medical treatment for hyperlipidemia can be accomplished with these factors in mind, while simultaneously following a ten-step geriatric patient prescribing process noted in Table 7.1.

In reviewing the "Ten Steps," it is evident that most medications used for treatment of hyperlipidemia have many positive attributes, to include clinical indication and known benefits, predictable side effect profile, established pharmacokinetics, once-a-day therapy, and little likelihood of a prescribing cascade. It is also remarkable that none of the commonly used agents for treatment of hyperlipidemia is included in the Beers Criteria as medications that are inappropriate for use in older adults [8].

Table 7.1 Ten steps to reduce polypharmacy in elderly patients

1. Obtain a complete history of ALL medications and supplements at each visit.
2. Use generic instead of trade names for each medication.
3. Review current medical problems. Is each medication still needed?
4. Use electronic prescribing tools to obtain information on drug interactions and side effects.
5. Consider modifying drug doses based on pharmacokinetic changes in drug metabolism due to normal aging.
6. Be ready to stop medications that are no longer indicated.
7. Review new clinical trial evidence and stop medications proven to be harmful (e.g., Stop hormone replacement in elderly women).
8. Choose medications with the lowest toxicity and highest safety (e.g., select inhaled nasal steroids instead of oral antihistamines for allergic rhinitis in elderly men).
9. Minimize prescribing medications to treat the side effects of another medication (e.g., prescribing proton-pump inhibitors to treat NSAID caused dyspepsia).
10. Select drugs with once-daily dosing and attempt to treat clinical conditions with a single medication.

Source: Adapted from Carlson, J. Perils of Polypharmacy: 10 steps to prudent prescribing. Geriatrics. 1996;51:26–35.

Treatment Risk Paradox

The phenomenon of inadequate treatment for those at increased age or risk of disease has been described by numerous authors. Referencing these studies and others, the study by Ko et al. on the "treatment–risk" paradox of lipid-lowering therapy with statins for high-risk older adults is particularly relevant to consider [9].

The elderly have the greatest baseline risk for cardiovascular disease. Ko's retrospective cohort study of elderly residents of Ontario showed that only 19.1% of elderly patients with cardiovascular disease and or diabetes received statins for secondary prevention of disease. Patients with diabetes, congestive heart failure, stroke, or lower socioeconomic status were also less likely to be prescribed a statin. Ko et al. pointed out that "For each year of increase in age and each 1% increase in the baseline risk index, there was a 6.4% lower odds of statin prescription...after adjustment for all other factors." This research points to an overall "emphasis of harm combined with an under-appreciation of benefits" that results in a "conservative hands-off approach to treatment" [9]. Other factors that may contribute to this paradox include misconceptions of benefit–harm tradeoffs, prejudgment of compliance by physicians (caused by cognitive, functional, and social decline), physician inattentiveness to cardiovascular prevention, and negative perception of benefits by patients [9].

A follow-up study on older (age, 60–75 years) male participants of the British Regional Heart Study noted a similar phenomenon of limited use of lipid-lowering medications in elderly patients with diagnoses of myocardial infarction (MI) and angina [10]. Of the 286 participants with a history of MI, 36% (102) were taking a lipid lowering medication (93 of the 102 were taking a statin). Among 360 men with angina without MI, 23% were taking a lipid-lowering agent (78 or 84 taking a statin). More than 80% of those individuals with established CHD had total cholesterol concentrations in excess of 5 mmol/l (193 mg/dl). Fewer than half of the patients receiving an agent for therapy met cholesterol-lowering goals, and only one-third of patients on statins were receiving trial-validated doses.

Prevention Strategies in the Elderly

When discussing prevention strategies and outcomes of therapy for geriatric patients, individualizing the care is paramount. Recent life expectancy studies demonstrate that an average 65-year-old has 18.4 years of additional life expectancy. At the age of 85, the average American has 6.8 years of additional life expectancy. Although statin therapy may seem unreasonable in a patient with end-stage lung disease or metastatic cancer, statin therapy appears more beneficial in a vital, community-dwelling 70-year-old with coronary artery disease (CAD) or CAD risk factors.

Evidence

Studies of Older Patients with Coronary Artery Disease (Secondary Prevention Studies) (Table 7.2)

Scandinavian Simvastatin Survival Study (4S)

Three important findings are remarkable in this secondary prevention trial [11] of treatment of patients with existing CHD. First, the amount of lipid change was similar between age cohorts. Second, absolute reductions in all-cause mortality were much more evident in the elderly population. Third, safety and tolerability profiles were similar across age cohorts.

The LIPID (Long-Term Intervention with Pravistatin in Ischaemic Disease) Study

The results of the LIPID Trial reemphasized the importance of age as being a major independent risk factor for CAD events [11]. Greater benefit in terms of absolute risk reduction was demonstrated in the older age cohort with resultant favorable numbers needed to treat (NNT of 22 for all-cause mortality in the older cohort versus 46 for the younger cohort). There was no difference in adverse reactions between age cohorts.

Heart Protection Study

The Heart Protection Study (HPS) included more than 2592 patients with diabetes over the age of 65. An additional 4063 patients over the age of 65 with known CAD (but without diabetes) were also enrolled. Simvastatin recipients of both groups noted significant reductions in coronary events, stroke, revascularization, and major coronary events [12].

Studies of Geriatric Age Patients Without CAD (Primary Prevention Studies)

AFCAPS/TEXCAPS Study

This primary prevention study of men and women involved 1416 patients over the age of 65. Similar reductions in lipid parameters were noted, with no significant

Table 7.2 Secondary prevention trials in the elderly

Trial	Type	Agent	Number of patients older than 65 in active arm	Duration	Cholesterol reduction	Cardiovascular (CV) endpoints
4S	DBPC	Simvastatin	1021 patients; age 65–70 years	Mean, 5.4 years	25% in TC 35% in LDL 10% in TG	34% decrease in ACM 43% decrease in CAD mortality 34% decrease in MCA 33% decrease in NFMI 34% decrease in other endpoints 41% decrease in revascularization 28% reduction in stroke and TIA
LIPID Trial	DBPC	Pravastatin (40 mg)	1741 patients; age 65–75 years	Mean 6.1 years	19% in TC 28% in LDL 7% increase in HDL 11% in TG	21% decrease ACM (NNT = 22) 24% decrease in CAD mortality (NNT = 28) 26% reduction MI (NNT = 30) 12% decrease in stroke (NS) 34% decrease in PTCA (NNT = 112) 26% decrease in CABG (NNT = 40)
CARE	DBPC	Pravastatin (40 mg)	1283	Median, 5 years	20% in TC 32% in LDL 5% increase in HDL 14% in TG	45% decrease in CAD death (NNT = 22) 39% decrease in CAD death or NFMI (NNT = 15) 32% decrease coronary events (NNT = 11) 32% decrease in revascularization 40% decrease in stroke 23% decrease in CHF 8% decrease in angina pectoris
HPS	DBPC (mixed primary and secondary prevention study)	Simvastatin (40 mg)	2592 diabetics over the age of 65; 5105 patients over the age of 65 with known arterial occlusive disease	5 years	TC and LDL 34% each	Diabetic patients: 27% reduction coronary events 20% reduction coronary mortality 37% reduction in first NFMI 24% reduction in first stroke 17% reduction in revascularization

Table 7.2 (continued)

Trial	Type	Agent	Number of patients older than 65 in active arm	Duration	Cholesterol reduction	Cardiovascular (CV) endpoints
ALLHAT-LLT	Randomized nonblinded; mixed primary and secondary prevention study	Pravastatin (40 mg/day)	2859	4.8 years, with follow-up for up to 8 years	17% in TC 28% in LDL 3% increase in HDL	Nondiabetic patients: 27% reduction in coronary events 26% reduction in first stroke 26% reduction in revascularization No significant reduction in all-cause mortality and CHD outcomes
PROSPER	DBPC	Pravastatin (40 mg/day)	1306 (mean age, 75.4 years)	3.2 years	34% in LDL 5% increase in HDL 12% in TG	19% reduction in NFMI 24% reduction in CHD death No reduction in stroke risk
SPARCL	DBPC	Atorvastatin (80 mg/day)	Mean age, 63 years	4.9 years	33% in TC 53% in LDL 23% in TG	16% reduction in stroke 23% reduction in stroke or TIA 35% reduction in coronary events 49% reduction in NFMI

Source: Data from Hunt D, Young P, Simes J, Hague W, Mann S, Owensby D, Lane G, Tonkin A. Benefits of pravastatin on cardiovascular events and mortality in older patients with coronary heart disease are equal to or exceed those seen in younger patients: results from the LIPID Trial. Ann Intern Med 2001;134:931–940; Collins R et al. MRC/BHF Heart Protection Study of cholesterol-lowering with simvastatin in 5963 people with diabetes: a randomised placebo-controlled trial. Lancet 2003;361:2005–2016. Colhoun HM, Betteridge DJ, Durrington PN, et al., on behalf of the CARDS Investigators. Primary prevention of cardiovascular disease with atorvastatin in type 2 diabetes in the Collaborative Atorvastatin Diabetes Study (CARDS): multicentre randomised pacebo-controlled trial. Lancet 2004;364:685–696; Shepherd J, Blauw GJ, Murphy M, et al., on behalf of the PROSPER study group. Pravastatin in elderly individuals at risk of vascular disease (PROSPER): a randomised controlled trial. Lancet 2002;360:1623–30; Shepherd J, Blauw GJ, Murphy M, et al., on behalf of the PROSPER study group. Preventing the next event in the elderly: the PROSPER perspective. Atherosclerosis Suppl 2003;4:17–22.

differences between the younger and older cohorts. Clinical prevention endpoints were all statistically better in the treatment group [13].

The CARDS Trial

This unique primary prevention trial demonstrated beneficial effect of atorvastatin on prevention of first occurrence of acute CHD events and stroke among patients with type 2 diabetes who had no preceding evidence of cardiovascular disease and without high LDL cholesterol. Of the atorvastatin recipients, 870 were over the age of 60, with a mean age of the study population being 61.5 years. Again, there were no differences of effect or hazard between the younger and older age cohorts [14].

The Special Nature of the PROSPER Study

This study randomized 5804 individuals from age 70 to 82 years and is unique among the statin prevention trials in that it examined the effects of statins exclusively in the elderly. The study enrolled both individuals with preexisting vascular disease (2565 or 44% of the study population) and those without (3239 or 56% of the study population). Pravastatin use led to a 19% reduction in coronary events but had no significant effect on cerebrovascular events. The risk for CHD death was significantly reduced by 24% in the pravastatin group. With an overall 2.1% absolute reduction in the primary endpoint, the PROSPER author notes that it would be necessary to treat 48 patients per year to avert one cardiac event [15].

This benefit (and evident lack of harm) was present in the face of considerable polypharmacy, with as many as 16 different drugs being taken by members of the pravastatin treatment arms. Overall, the PROSPER data "extends to elderly individuals the treatment strategy currently used in middle aged people" [16].

Stroke

Statin prevention of cerebrovascular disease has been addressed in a variety of trials, as already noted. What is suggested by the data is that cerebrovascular benefit may not develop until after 5 to 6 years of therapy.

Cost-Effectiveness of Therapy in the Elderly

The age-related demographic changes in the decades to come, coupled with age-associated vascular diseases, implies significant individual and societal burden will occur. The role that lipid-lowering agents (particularly statins) may play in reducing this burden is seriously debated, especially in treatment of the aged.

To date, the studies of statin use in older patients demonstrate event reduction similar to younger participants, to include early benefit for CHD reduction and stroke benefit with longer courses of therapy. Also, studies support the concept that treatment with statins is most effective as the baseline risk in an individual increases, not a preset number for total cholesterol and LDL.

A more recent study looking at cost-effectiveness of treatment of older individuals aged 65 to 75 years compared to younger patients was completed by Australian researchers. The authors concluded that the incremental cost per life saved was $41,400 in older adults and $124,700 in younger patients. The concluding remark from this analysis is worth repeating: "Cholesterol-lowering therapy with 3-hydroxy-3-methylglutaryl co-enzyme A reductase inhibitors should be generally available and very widely prescribed in older patients with CHD. The attitude of physicians who may withhold therapy in the elderly because of their shorter life expectancy should change, and measures to support compliance with treatment should be implemented [17]".

Summary

CHD is the most common cause of death in the elderly, and that risk increases with aging. Life expectancy for the elderly is increasing, and for many with CHD and cerebrovascular disease risk factors, statin therapy during their remaining years of life likely offers morbidity and mortality benefit. The evidence now strongly supports the protective benefits in secondary prevention and confers primary prevention benefit when vascular disease risk factors (diabetes, hypertension, metabolic syndrome) are present.

The role of statin therapy in those over the age of 85 is currently debated. It would seem reasonable to continue therapy if faced with a need for secondary prevention and to reconsider therapy in the absence of comorbidities in this age group.

Drug therapy for this group can be safely initiated because of the favorable and predictable side effect profile of these agents. Cost of medical therapy is a potentially significant burden for the elderly, but this can be mitigated by generic availability and Medicare drug benefits for elders in need.

Women

Cardiovascular disease is the chief killer of women as well as men. Although men tend to develop cardiovascular disease at a younger age, the annual number of deaths from cardiovascular disease in women exceeds that of men. Furthermore, although mortality from cardiovascular disease has decreased in men over the last 30 years, this has not been true to the same extent in women [18]. Yet, the past decade has led to more insights into the unique clinical presentation of coronary disease in women as well as someof the issues that are unique in developing an evidence-based prevention strategy for an individual woman patient.

The early statin trials included only 15% to 20% women. Subsequent meta-analyses of these trials have confirmed that statins reduce events as much in women as in men, with slightly more strokes prevented than heart attacks. The American

Heart Association (AHA) released evidence-based guidelines for cardiovascular disease prevention in women for the first time in 2004 [19]. These provide an excellent starting point for making recommendations on the treatment of hyperlipidemia in women.

The first step is to determine the individual cardiovascular risk status of a woman to help determine the required intensity of therapy. Although the use of the Framingham Risk factor tool (see Chapter 2) is encouraged, it is important to recognize that this tool can underestimate risk in women. There is a growing body of literature supporting the use of adjunctive screening tools in women. In particular, high-sensitivity C-reactive protein (hs-crp) has a high level of usefulness for risk assessment in women who are considered to be at intermediate risk by traditional Framingham assessment [20].

A program of therapeutic lifestyle changes is then initiated to include smoking cessation, 30 min of physical activity on most days, weight management to maintain

Table 7.3 Cardiovascular risk factor interventions in women

Risk factor	Intervention	Level of evidence
Blood pressure greater than 140/90 mm Hg[a]	Pharmacotherapy	A
LDL greater than 100 mg/dl	Lifestyle and pharmacotherapy with a statin based on target LDL level per NCEP guidelines	A
HDL greater than 50 mg/dl	Lifestyle and pharmacotherapy with niacin or a fibrate to raise HDL	B
TG greater than 150 mg/d	Lifestyle and pharmacotherapy with a fibrate or niacin to lower TG	B
Elevated blood glucose or HBA1C	Lifestyle or pharmacotherapy to maintain normal blood glucose and HBA1C below 7.0%	A/B
Thrombosis	Aspirin therapy (75–162 mg/day) should be considered in all women at intermediate or high risk	A
Menopause	Estrogen and/or progesterone therapy should not be initiated, or continued to prevent cardiovascular disease	A
Postmyocardial infarction	Beta-blockers should be used indefinitely	A
Heart failure or an ejection fraction less than 40%	ACE inhibitors should be prescribed unless contraindicated; ARBs should be used in women intolerant of ACE inhibitors	A/B

ARBs, angiotensin II receptor blockers; ACE inhibitor, angiotensin-converting enzyme inhibitor
[a]Cutoff for treatment is lower in the presence of diabetes or target organ damage.
Source: Data from Mosca L, Appel LJ, Benjamin EJ, et al. Evidence based guidelines for cardiovascular disease prevention in women. Circulation 2004;109:672–693.

a BMI between 18.5 and 24.9 kg/m [2] and a waist circumference less than 35 in., a heart-healthy diet (see Chapter 3), and treatment for depression when clinically indicated.

Next, cardiovascular risk-reducing interventions are recommended based on the risk status of a patient. A summary of these risk factor interventions is outlined in Table 7.3.

Adults Younger Than 35 Years of Age

Statin trials have largely excluded patients younger than 35 years of age because of the low likelihood of cardiovascular events in this age group. As a result, any decisions to treat men and women less than 35 years of age are based primarily on clinical extrapolation and not trial evidence. Additionally, although family history of premature atherosclerotic cardiovascular disease (ASCVD) is very predictive of events in patients under 45 years of age, the Framingham risk criteria do not account for family history when assigning a risk category. Therefore, young patients at a high genetic risk can have a falsely reassuring low risk of disease based solely on a Framingham calculation.

Although clinical trial data are sparse, epidemiologic evidence is strong. Autopsy studies from men killed in Vietnam showed advanced atherosclerotic lesions in soldiers as young as 18 years of age. These soldiers almost always had a family history significant for coronary death in male relatives before the age of 50. The Bogalusa Heart Study, the Muscatine Study, and the Pathobiologic Determinants of Atherosclerosis in Youth (PDAY) studies form another large part of this epidemiologic evidence [21–23].

These long-term studies provide the evidence that atherosclerosis is a largely predictable process that begins in childhood as early as age 2 and progresses at a rate determined by coronary risk factors. It is accelerated or decelerated by the accumulation or reduction of these risk factors [21–23]. Coronary artery risk factors in children and adolescents are associated with the early development of atherosclerosis in adults: these include low HDL, high BMI, high blood pressure, and high LDL. Startlingly, the carotid intima medial thickness (IMT) of adults (a surrogate for systemic atherosclerosis) can be predicted by *childhood* measures of LDL and BMI [24].

The implications of this epidemiologic information are that early intervention will likely slow atherosclerosis. However, there are no prospective trials proving better outcomes with an early initiation of lipid reduction therapy. In fact, it is likely that there will never be results from such trials, which would require thousands of patients and last for decades at a tremendous cost. It is also important to remember that the number-needed-to-treat (NNT) for a patient under the age of 35 can be as high as 250:1, making a treatment decision very costly compared to the treatment of an elderly patient, in which the NNT can be as low as 4:1.

What then is a reasonable approach to the primary prevention of ASCVD in patients under 35? The ATP III (Adult Treatment Panel, National Cholesterol

Education Panel) helps to strike a middle ground by stating that although clinically significant atherosclerotic disease is rare in the young, atherosclerosis can progress rapidly in young adults so that pharmacologic treatment may be advisable for young patients who have LDL greater than 190 mg/dl or who smoke and have LDL greater than 160 mg/dl.

The preferred approach of this author is to begin aggressive therapeutic lifestyle changes (TLC) for all young patients at high risk of ASCVD based on traditional risk assessment, with additional strong consideration of any family history of atherosclerotic disease under the age of 50. Aggressive TLC means helping the patient to avoid smoking, to maintain a BMI under 25 kg/m [2] through a heart-healthy diet, to participate in an exercise program that has at least 30 min of moderate physical activity on 5 to 7 days of the week, to increase consumption of soluble fiber, and to drink one glass of red wine with dinner for those who consume alcohol. For those patients who continue to have an LDL greater than 160 mg/dl or an HDL less than 30 mg/dl despite aggressive TLC, the use of a statin or niacin is offered to the patients. Therapy is individualized based on the patient's desires and risk.

Children

Risk factors measured in youth are predictive of accelerated atherosclerosis in adulthood. The optimum time to create healthy lifestyle habits is in childhood before unhealthy habits become ingrained. Because most lipid-lowering medications are not formally U.S. Food and Drug Administration (FDA) approved for use in children, lifestyle interventions are crucial, which adds a further challenge to clinical decisions in the care of patients under the age of 18. As noted earlier in this chapter, the epidemiologic and physiological evidence is strong that atherosclerosis begins as early as age 2 and progresses at a rate determined by both a patient's individual genetic predisposition and the presence of other risk factors such as smoking, diabetes, obesity, and hypertension. No child should have their lipid levels checked before the age of 2 because elevated lipids are normal from birth to 24 months.

Resins are safe and approved for use in children. However, compliance with resins is very poor in children, who are unlikely to tolerate the frequent gastrointestinal side effects. Similarly, most children who are considered for treatment have familial dyslipidemia syndromes with LDL cholesterols greater than 200 to 300 mg/dl. Statins are the only class of medications with the potency to reduce these LDL values closer to a less risky range.

The "normal" range for lipids is also less clear in children. The National Cholesterol Education Program (NCEP) last issued a guideline on lipids in children in 1992 [25]. The cutoff value for a high LDL cholesterol was set at 130 mg/dl largely based on expert opinion and not extensive demographic information. Only recently, in 2006, have investigators published the normal distribution of lipoproteins by age and gender in adolescents. This study developed lipoprotein curves akin to growth curves that give clinicians the ability to interpret an adolescent's lipid profile in comparison to age and gender means and extremes [26].

Several trials in the last decade have given a growing evidence base to the use of statins in patients from 8 to 18 years of age [27,28]. At present, simvastatin and atorvastatin have been studied and appear safe in children from 10 to 17 years of age. Pravastatin has been studied in children from 8 to 18 years of age and appears effective and safe as well. The main safety concern with statins has to do with their use before menarche and pubarche. One reasonable approach is to optimize aggressive TLC (as noted earlier in this chapter) until pubarche and then consider the use of statins after that point.

The American Heart Association (AHA) guidelines for the prevention of atherosclerosis beginning in childhood reinforce the need to screen all children after the age of 2 who have family histories of premature cardiovascular disease [29]. The AHA uses the 1992 NCEP guidelines of an LDL greater than 110 mg/dl as borderline and an LDL greater than 130 mg/dl as elevated. Lifestyle changes are encouraged for all, and pharmacologic intervention is considered with resins or statins for children with high-risk family histories and LDL greater than 160 mg/dl despite lifestyle changes [29].

It is also important to recognize that lifestyle changes in children require lifestyle changes in *the adults who care for them*. Effective diet and exercise counseling must be aimed at the parents as well as the children. If the adult caretakers of the children smoke, they must be enrolled in smoking cessation classes because one of the strongest predictors of adolescent smoking is exposure to parents who smoke. Effective lifestyle changes are optimized when the entire family unit is engaged in change versus a single at-risk child.

Native Americans

It is well known that Native Americans suffer from rates of cardiovascular morbidity and mortality that are higher than the U.S. population means. The multiyear Strong Heart Study has studied Native American populations in 13 different communities for decades and has helped to form a better understanding of the unique risk factors that contribute to this increased rate of cardiovascular disease (CVD) [30].

CVD morbidity and mortality were similar in all communities but more than two times higher than those seen in a large population study of non-Native Americans. It was noted that despite the decline in CVD rates in non-Native Americans, the rates in Native Americans were increasing. The investigators attributed this risk primarily to a much greater incidence of diabetes, not to abnormally high rates of dyslipidemia or hypertension.

In fact, other studies have shown that a larger proportion of Native Americans have desirable cholesterol levels of less than 200 mg/dl and fewer had high triglyceride (TG) levels greater than 240 mg/dl than non-Native Americans [31]. The Strong Heart Study also showed that despite the greater rates of CVD, mean TC was 20 mg/dl lower in men and 27 mg/dl lower in women than compared to national means. Mean HDL levels were also higher among Native Americans as compared to national means [32].

The ramifications of this for clinicians caring for Native Americans is that despite lipid profiles that are more favorable than the average U.S. population, rates of diabetes are much higher. Risk assessment should include a focus on diabetes screening as well. LDL goals should be similar in Native Americans or non-Native Americans. Patients with diabetes should have an LDL goal of less than 100 mg/dl, with an optional goal of less than 70 mg/dl if they have other risk factors for CVD.

Elite Athletes

Because exercise benefits an individual by having a positive effect on their serum lipids, it stands to reason that elite athletes should have lipid panels that are considered excellent or at least better than sedentary controls. It should also be true that elite athletes have a lower-than-average risk for cardiovascular disease.

Definition of an Elite Athlete

Elite athletes are by definition special. They may be club-level athletes, college athletes, professional athletes, or local athletes who train hard and excel during competition. They are a small dominant group within the larger population of athletes who are well respected by our society at large for the commitment they make to their sport. It goes without saying that elite athletes train harder than what is expected for "regular" athletes. Physiologically, elite athletes push their own limits, often to the point of injury or organ dysfunction.

Lipid Subfractions

Total cholesterol (TC) and LDL cholesterol are generally unaffected by exercise. Extreme exertion can lead to a 5% decrease in LDL cholesterol. In contrast, even small amounts of regular exercise will decrease TG and increase HDL by up to 50%. Therefore, when interpreting the lipid profile of an elite athlete, it is important to recognize that TG and HDL values should be different than what is considered normal compared to a population mean.

High HDL levels have been consistently demonstrated in elite athletes when compared to their sedentary counterparts. On average, HDL levels are 10 to 20 mg/dl (40%–50%) higher than sedentary control levels. Some studies have even been able to demonstrate a difference in HDL levels across different sport types. There may be a higher potential to increase HDL levels with endurance or aerobic-type sports as compared to power sports or those that are primarily anaerobic. In one study, primarily speed athletes (sprinters) or anaerobic athletes (e.g., power lifters) had similar or even lower HDL levels than their matched sedentary controls [33]. This advantage has not been consistently shown to be the case, however. In one study comparing Olympic athletes to sedentary age-matched medical students, primarily anaerobic athletes (power lifters) showed levels of HDL above that of the controls. Overall, athletes in the latter study had better serum lipid parameters than sedentary controls, and their HDL levels correlated to their VO_2 max and relative body weight.

The Effect of Anabolic Steroids on Lipids

Competitive athletics is the major world stage in which use of anabolic steroids is regularly discovered. The perceived benefits of anabolic steroids (increased muscle mass, improved performance) are tempting to athletes who desire to play themselves into the elite of their sport. Recently, numerous Major League Baseball and National Football League players have failed drug tests for anabolic steroid use.

Anabolic steroids have detrimental effects on serum lipids [34]. Glazer described a decrease in HDL levels by 39% to 70% with anabolic steroid use as determined by meta-analysis. An increase in LDL levels by 11% to 100%, with a mean increase of 36% from baseline, was noted [35]. Overall, high-dose anabolic steroids lower HDL, increase LDL, and increase atherogenic-promoting apolipoproteins. The detrimental morbidity and mortality caused by cardiovascular events are unclear, but all changes in serum lipids seen with anabolic steroid use have proven to be atherogenic in humans [36]. Most of the effects occur acutely and can regress with cessation of steroid use over 3 to 5 weeks.

Female Elite Athletes

Female athletes who train and compete at an elite level have special concerns with regard to reproductive potential, bone density, and mental health. In general, the effect of serum estrogen in women has allowed for an overall better lipid profile and reduced risk of coronary disease while premenopausal. Reduced estrogen levels in women can occur with dietary limitation and excessive exercise. The female athlete triad is one condition known to result when a negative caloric balance occurs.

Female Athlete Triad

Female athletes who exercise regularly and to an extreme may notice a change in menstrual cycles. These women are at particularly high risk of disordered eating, which includes hypocaloric intake for what is necessary for their specific energy output. Bone health suffers in these women, and they can demonstrate osteopenia or frank osteoporosis late in the course of the condition. Bone health deterioration is often the first recognized sign of the triad as an athlete is sidelined from a stress fracture. Often a stress fracture in a female athlete leads to an evaluation to discover if the female athletic triad exists.

The triad refers to a patient who experiences amenorrhea, osteoporosis, and an eating disorder. There may be slight variations in severity of each arm of the triad (i.e., oligomenorrhea instead of amenorrhea, osteopenia instead of osteoporosis, disordered eating instead of a full-blown disorder). Extreme exercise and dietary limitation lead to dysfunction of the hypothalamic-pituitary-ovarian axis, which is responsible for regulating the production of sex hormones in women. The athlete becomes estrogen deficient, and serum lipids deteriorate as well.

In a study of athletes who were amenorrheic compared with those who exercised similarly but had normal or oligomenorrheic cycles, the amenorrheic patients had significantly higher total cholesterol and LDL levels. The levels were both above normal levels [37]. The long-term cardiovascular risk in these athletes has not yet been elucidated.

Considerations in the Treatment of Elite Athletes with Dyslipidemia

As with nonathletic populations, elite athletes with dyslipidemia significant enough to need medication are likely to be prescribed a statin-type drug to control their serum lipids. Statins have become the cornerstone of medical lipid management, in large part because of their effectiveness and tolerability.

Concerns exist regarding use of statins with elite athletes. One potential side effect of the stain class is symptomatic muscle aches and cramps. Elevated creatinine kinase (CK) levels from the medication have been seen and may be of particular concern in athletes, as their high exertion puts them at risk of muscle damage and rises in CK levels independent of their statin therapy. Dehydration is often seen in athletics and may exacerbate the rise in CK and the potential for rhabdomyolysis. Rhabdomyolysis has been seen following extreme exertion and may be more common with statin drug use.

No studies have definitively evaluated the use of statins during extreme exertion. However, a prudent rule is that statins should be withheld 1 week before extreme endurance events (ultramarathons, ironman competitions, eco-challenges, etc.), because profound intracompetition dehydration can increase the risk of rhabdomyolysis.

Detraining Effects

Exercise clearly increases HDL and reduces TG in elite endurance athletes. If the training ceases, these positive effects on the serum lipid panel tend to reverse. In a case-control study of 20 athletes of the effects of detraining on lipids, 10 of the athletes trained for 2 years an average of 22 h per week. The other 10 trained similarly for 1 year and then stopped. Following detraining at 1 year, HDL decreased by 19%, TG increased by 49%, and LDL increased by 13%.

During the study, participants exercised for 47 weeks and then had a 5-week detraining phase. Detraining produced a rapid loss of endurance training benefits in serum lipids. The changes in serum lipids (for the worse) began to occur after only 5 weeks of detraining. This finding leads to the suspicion that highly trained athletes who detrain abruptly may be at risk of cardiovascular disease shortly after changing their exertion levels.

Summary

Elite athletes should have TG and HDL levels well above the desired ATP III values of less than 150 mg/dl and greater than 40 mg/dl, respectively. When assessing cardiovascular risk in athletes, it is important to expect a lipid profile better than population means and to think about substances that are ingested to improve performance. The potential negative effects of extreme exercise on women through the female athlete triad must also be considered. Lipid abnormalities that exist despite vigorous exercise should be treated. Statins should be withheld 1 week before extreme endurance events (ultramarathons, ironman competitions, eco-challenges, etc.), because intracompetition dehydration can increase the risk of rhabdomyolysis.

The Patient with Multiple Medical Problems

In addressing the role that medical management of hyperlipidemia may play in the treatment of a patient with multiple medical problems, the clinician must apply the art of medicine and the science of evidence-based practice to the individual circumstance of each patient.

The decision to start therapy for hyperlipidemia is based on a multitude of factors, not just the type of changes in lipid profile and the goals of therapy. More fundamental and in some ways implicit questions are posed. Will my patient live for the next 2 to 5 years to derive benefit from the treatment? Does my patient have some condition that will result in death despite treatment of hyperlipidemia? Does my patient have severe liver or renal disease that prohibits treatment? Does my patient require treatment with some other agent that directly interacts with my choices?

Layered onto the clinician's decision-making process are the patient's knowledge, behaviors, and agenda that may reduce or add friction to management decisions. For example, the middle-aged male with newly diagnosed CAD may view his disease as "the family curse" and may balk at the cost and potential side effects of therapy because he perceives the "inevitability" of untimely death. Successful treatment in this context would be more focused on allying with the patient to reduce friction, exchange information, and promote attitudinal and behavioral change. With this task completed, treatment may be more successfully initiated.

After the initial risk assessment and agenda setting, the clinician must firmly establish if the therapeutic effort is driven by primary or secondary prevention and must communicate the goal to the patient. Secondary prevention with lipid-lowering therapy is often the easier "sell" after the patient's first heart attack, rather than the "tough sell" of primary prevention of behavioral change and medical therapy.

Viewing every clinic visit as an opportunity to reduce friction and to exchange information to promote wellness and prevention is an attitudinal approach for the clinician to consider.

As outlined in previous sections, polypharmacy poses a significant but not insurmountable barrier to initiating lipid-lowering therapy. Some general measures to consider:

- Adjusting dose based on renal and hepatic function
- Having detailed knowledge of all medications, supplements, and OTC medications
- Providing the patient a "do not take this medication if you take any of the following medications" list
- Starting only one new medication at a time
- Considering real versus perceived patient literacy skills to enhance safe patient compliance with therapy
- Considering clinical pharmacist review of the patient's medication and problem lists
- Promoting patient use of medication organizers, especially for nighttime use of statins
- Using electronic medical records or personal data assistants (PDAs) with software to conduct assessments for drug–drug interactions
- Enlisting family members as appropriate to assist in medication/diet/exercise compliance
- Celebrating success with your patient

The Patient with Atherosclerotic Cardiovascular Disease (ASCVD)

Treatment of hyperlipidemia as secondary prevention for patients with established ASCVD or CAD equivalent [diabetes, stroke, transient ischemic attack (TIA), atherosclerotic peripheral disease (ASPVD)] is well established in the literature. As previously described, treatment strategies to reduce LDL to less than 70 mg/dl is perhaps ideal, along with strategies to raise HDL and minimize triglyceride levels. Clinical trials suggest that fewer than half of all patient achieved LDL cholesterol goals with the starting dose of a statin, but more than 70% were never titrated, resulting in 45% of patients failing to reach ATP III goals [38]. In summary, the clinician needs to treat, reevaluate, titrate as necessary, and change agents or add an agent to achieve ATP III goals for prevention of subsequent events.

The decision to advise a patient on primary prevention begins with knowledge of the ATP III goals and patient risk factors and communicating those risk factors in terms that the patient can understand. Clinical practice suggests that risk communication is a very effective tool in the communication of primary prevention strategies. Generally speaking, an individual with zero or one risk factor has a 10-year mortality risk of less than 10%, with drug therapy consideration at LDL of 160 mg/dl in this individual. Further drug therapy decisions based upon patient risk factors and LDL are discussed elsewhere in this volume.

Primary drug–drug or drug–condition interactions to look for in this population are with warfarin, digoxin, verapamil, amiodarone (with statins), diuretics and propranolol with bile acid sequestrants or resins (BAS), oral hypoglycemics, and insulin (with fibrates). Any combination therapy with lipid-lowering agents should be monitored carefully for myopathy and liver toxicity.

The Patient with Atherosclerotic Peripheral Disease (ASPVD)

The treatment of hyperlipidemia in patients with ASPVD has been shown to be effective at reducing complications of this disease but requires longer duration of therapy (5 years or greater) to demonstrate full clinical benefit. Treatment strategies for ASCVD and ASPVD are complementary in that patients derive benefit from lipid-lowering therapy, anticoagulation, risk factor modification, and appropriate diet and exercise. Potential drug–drug and drug–condition interactions between lipid-lowering agents and agents for treatment of ASPVD are similar to those encountered in the treatment of ASCVD. To date, definitive data to support the use of lipid-lowering therapy as a primary prevention measure for ASPVD are limited.

The Patient with Dementia (Alzheimer's, Vascular, or Mixed Dementia)

Dementia is a heterogeneous disease, largely of the elderly, with 50% of dementias reflecting the degeneration of Alzheimer's disease (AD) and the remaining largely associated with cerebrovascular disease. Many researchers see underlying vascular pathology in degenerative dementias such as AD. The next problem is establishing a meaningful baseline for cognitive function, followed by using a sensitive clinical tool that is clinically relevant. (Just because a test result is significant does not mean that the result is relevant or meaningful.) The largest prospective study of this question was the PROSPER study, which failed to show any significant effect of pravastatin on cognitive function, a finding shared by the Heart Protection Study [12,15].

Medications commonly associated with dementia treatments (primarily acetyl cholinesterase inhibitors) are not strongly associated with drug–drug interactions with lipid lowering agents (MICROMEDEX 2006).

The Patient with Diabetes

The protective benefits of treating hyperlipidemia with lipid-lowering agents are well established, particularly with statins and fibrates, from both a primary and secondary prevention point of view. Diabetic patients, with their tendency to develop dense LDL molecules, may require more aggressive therapy to achieve desired goals and prevention of vascular injury. Considerations in the treatment of hyperlipidemia in diabetic patients are the potential risk of slight worsening of glucose control with niacin and rare hypoglycemic episodes associated with fibrates.

The Patient with Chronic Obstructive Pulmonary Disease (COPD)

Statins have no role in the direct therapy of chronic obstructive pulmonary disease (COPD). There are no evident drug–drug or disease–drug interactions between common COPD-related medications and lipid-lowering agents. No studies suggest benefit of lipid-lowering therapy for this condition.

The Patient with Chronic Infectious Disease

Drug interactions are possible when treating patients on lipid-lowering therapy. Altered lipid profiles are common in human immunodeficiency virus (HIV) patients as a side effect of the agents used to control the disease. Protease inhibitors block the metabolism pathways of many statins, increasing the circulating level of statins and increasing the risk of rhabdomyolysis. Agents with this interaction include simvastatin, lovastatin, and atorvastatin. Alternative agents for lipid-lowering therapy are advised in this situation such as niacin or resins.

Another potential for drug–drug interactions includes simultaneous treatment with azole antifungals (itraconazole and ketoconazole) and macrolides (erythromycin and others) and the statins atorvastatin, lovastatin, and simvastatin. These antifungals and antibiotics interact with the cytochrome P450 system and may result in increased levels of these statins, again resulting in myopathy. Dosage reduction or temporary statin discontinuation and careful monitoring are advised for the duration of antimicrobial therapy.

The Patient with Renal Disease

In general, patients with chronic kidney disease should be monitored closely when taking fibrates, with dose reductions based on level of disease. Monitoring of statin effects and dose changes based on the degree of kidney disease is also advised. BAS, niacin, and ezetimibe appear to require no additional significant renal monitoring.

The Patient with Liver Disease

Monitoring of hepatic enzymes and dosage adjustment is required for the following agents: statins, fibrates, niacin, and ezetimibe. Fulminant hepatic failure from statins is rare. Fibrates should not be used in patients with existing gallbladder disease. BAS should be discontinued in the presence of bowel obstruction.

The Frail Patient

Frailty is a loosely defined term usually applied to the aged that implies weight loss (nutritional compromise), weakness, executive dysfunction, and, often, dementia. Markers of this syndrome include loss of instrumental activities of daily living, weight loss, low serum albumin, low total cholesterol, and low total lymphocyte count (less than 1400). A risk-to-benefit assessment of continuation of lipid-lowering therapy should be performed in this clinical situation.

Family Issues

There are two key issues on which clinicians caring for patients with hyperlipidemia must focus. First, most elevated serum lipids are rooted in a genetically inherited predisposition. Therefore, the diagnosis of hyperlipidemia in one member of a family should prompt screening in all members of the family who have not been screened.

Second, the cornerstone of the treatment of hyperlipidemia is therapeutic lifestyle changes (TLC), which involves changes in diet, exercise, and modifiable risk factors such as smoking and obesity. TLC is most successful when the whole family is involved. If only one member of the family eats a heart-healthy diet and exercises daily, it is unlikely that this new lifestyle will take root for the long term. In contrast, when entire family units improve their eating habits, exercise regularly, and lose weight, a clinician is more likely to see long-term lifestyle changes that persist and significantly reduce the CVD risk in not just the initial patient, but the entire family unit. This multiplicative effect is the key to a larger population health impact in the reduction of unhealthy lifestyles and CVD risk.

References

1. Lerner DJ, Kanner WK. Patterns of coronary heart disease morbidity and mortality in the sexes: a 26 year follow-up of the Framingham population. Am Heart J 1986;111:383–390.
2. Merck Institute of Aging and Health. The state of aging and health in America 2004. Washington, DC: Merck Institute of Aging and Health (MIAH), 2004:1.
3. Katzel LI, Goldberg AP. Dyslipoproteinemia. In: Hazzard WR, Blass JP, Ettinger WH, et al. (eds) Principles of geriatric medicine and gerontology, 4th edn. New York: McGraw-Hill, 1999:1013–1028.
4. Beck L. Aging changes in renal function. In: Hazzard WR, Blass JP, Ettinger WH, et al. (eds) Principles of geriatric medicine and gerontology, 4th edn. New York: McGraw-Hill, 1999.
5. Weverling-Rijnsburger AW, Blauw GJ, Lagaay AM, et al. Total cholesterol and risk of mortality in the oldest old. Lancet 1997;350(9085):1119–1123.
6. Shipley MJ, Pocock SJ, Marmot MG. Does plasma cholesterol concentration predict mortality from coronary heart disease in elderly people? 18-year follow up in Whitehall study. BMJ 1991;303:89–92.
7. Fouts M, Hanlon J, Pieper C, et al. Identification of elderly nursing home residents at high risk for drug related problems. Consult Pharmacol 1997;12:1103–1111.

8. Fink DM, Cooper JW, Wade WE, et al. Updating the Beers criteria for potentially inappropriate medication use in older adults. Arch Intern Med 2003;163:2716–2722.
9. Ko DT, Mamdani M, Alter DA. Lipid-lowering therapy with statins in high-risk elderly patients: the treatment-risk paradox. JAMA 2004;291(15):1864–1870.
10. Whincup PH, Emberson JR, Lennon L, et al. Low prevalence of lipid lowering drug use in older men with established coronary heart disease. Heart 2002;88:25–29.
11. Hunt D, Young P, Simes J, et al. Benefits of pravastatin on cardiovascular events and mortality in older patients with coronary heart disease are equal to or exceed those seen in younger patients: results from the LIPID Trial. Ann Intern Med 2001;134:931–940.
12. Collins R, Armitage J, Parish S, Sleigh P, Peto R. Heart Protection Study Collaborative Group. MRC/BHF Heart Protection Study of cholesterol-lowering with simvastatin in 5963 people with diabetes: a randomised placebo-controlled trial. Lancet 2003;361:2005–2016.
13. Downs JR, Clearfield M, Weis S, et al., for the AFCAPS/TexCAPS Research Group. Primary prevention of acute coronary events with lovastatin in men and women with average cholesterol levels: results of AFCAPS/TexCAPS. JAMA 1998;279(20):1615–1622.
14. Colhoun HM, Betteridge DJ, Durrington PN, et al., on behalf of the CARDS Investigators. Primary prevention of cardiovascular disease with atorvastatin in type 2 diabetes in the Collaborative Atorvastatin Diabetes Study (CARDS): multicentre randomised placebo-controlled trial. Lancet 2004;364:685–696.
15. Shepherd J, Blauw GJ, Murphy M, et al., on behalf of the PROSPER study group. Pravastatin in elderly individuals at risk of vascular disease (PROSPER): a randomised controlled trial. Lancet 2002;360:1623–1630.
16. Shepherd J, Blauw GH, Murphy M, et al., on behalf of the PROSPER study group. Preventing the next event in the elderly: the PROSPER perspective. Atherosclerosis Suppl 2003;4:17–22.
17. Tonmin AM, Eckerman S, White H, et al. Cost effectiveness of cholesterol lowering therapy with pravastatin in patients with previous coronary syndromes aged 65 to 74 years compared with younger patients. Am Heart J 2006;151:1305–1312.
18. American Heart Association. Heart Disease and Stroke Statistics: 2005 Update. http://www.americanheart.org/presenter.jhtml?identifier=3000090. Accessed 07/07/06.
19. Mosca L, Appel LJ, Benjamin EJ, et al. Evidence based guidelines for cardiovascular disease prevention in women. Circulation 2004;109:672–693.
20. Ridker PM, Rifai N, Rose L, et al. Comparison of C-reactive protein and low-density lipoprotein cholesterol levels in the prediction of first cardiovascular events. N Engl J Med 2002;347:1557–1565.
21. Anonymous. Relationship of atherosclerosis in young men to serum lipoprotein cholesterol concentrations and smoking: a preliminary report from the Pathobiological Determinants of Atherosclerosis in Youth (PDAY) Research Group. JAMA 1990;264:3018–3024.
22. Mahoney LT, Burns TL, Stanford W, et al. Coronary risk factors measured in childhood and young adult life are associated with coronary artery calcification in young adults: the Muscatine Study. J Am Coll Cardiol 1996;27:277–284.
23. Berenson GS, Srinivasan SR, Bao W, et al. Association between multiple cardiovascular risk factors and atherosclerosis in children and young adults: the Bogalusa Heart Study. N Engl J Med 1998;338:1650–1656.
24. Li S, Chen W, Srinivasan SR, et al. Childhood cardiovascular risk factors and carotid vascular changes in adulthood. JAMA 2003;290:2271–2277.
25. NCEP. Highlights of the report of the expert panel on blood cholesterol levels in children and adolescents. Pediatrics 1992;89:495–501.
26. Jolliffe CJ, Janssen I. Distribution of lipoproteins by age and gender in adolescents. Circulation 2006;114:1056–1062.
27. Wiegman A, Hutten BA, de Groot E, et al. Efficacy and safety of statin therapy in children with familial hypercholesterolemia: a randomized controlled trial. JAMA 2004;292:331–337.

28. de Jongh S, Lilien MR, Op't Roodt J, et al. Early statin therapy restores endothelial function in children with familial hypercholesterolemia. J Am Coll Cardiol 2002;40:2117–2121.
29. Kavey REW, Daniels SR, Lauer RM, et al. AHA guidelines for primary prevention of atherosclerotic cardiovascular disease beginning in childhood. Circulation 2003;107: 1562–1566.
30. Howard BV, Lee ET, Cown LD, et al. Rising tide of cardiovascular disease in American Indians. The Strong Heart Study. Circulation 1999;99:2389–2395.
31. Robbins DC, Welty TK, Wang WY, et al. Plasma lipids and lipoprotein concentrations among American Indians: comparison with the US population. Curr Opin Lipidol 1996;7:188–195.
32. Welty TK, Lee ET, Yeh J, et al. Cardiovascular disease risk factors among American Indians: the Strong Heart Study. Am J Epidemiol 1995;142:269–287.
33. Wood P, Williams PT, Haskell WL. Physical activity and high density lipoproteins. In: Miller NE, Miller GJ (eds) Clinical and metabolic aspects of high density lipoproteins. Amsterdam: Elsevier, 1984:133–165.
34. Modlinski R, Fields KB. The effect of anabolic steroids on the gastrointestinal system, kidneys, and adrenal glands. Curr Sports Med Rep 2006;5(2):104–109.
35. Glazer G. Atherogenic effects of anabolic steroids on serum lipid levels. Arch Intern Med 1991;151:1925–1933.
36. Sullivan ML, Martinez CM, Gennis P, et al. The cardiac toxicity of anabolic steroids. Prog Cardiovasc Dis 1998;41:1–5.
37. Rickenlund A, Eriksson MJ, et al. Amenorrhea in female athletes is associated with endothelial dysfunction and unfavorable lipid profile. J Clin Endocrinol Metab 2005;90(3):1354–1359.
38. Crouse JR III, Elam MB, Robinson JG, et al. Cholesterol management: targeting a lower low density lipoprotein cholesterol concentration increases ATP-III goal attainment. Am J Cardiol 2006;97(11):1667–1669.

Suggested Key Readings

Berenson GS, Srinivasan SR, Bao W, et al. Association between multiple cardiovascular risk factors and atherosclerosis in children and young adults: the Bogalusa Heart Study. N Engl J Med 1998;338:1650–1656.
Kavey REW, Daniels SR, Lauer RM, et al. AHA Guidelines for primary prevention of atherosclerotic cardiovascular disease beginning in childhood. Circulation 2003;107:1562–1566.
Mosca L, Appel LJ, Benjamin EJ, et al. Evidence based guidelines for cardiovascular disease prevention in women. Circulation 2004;109:672–693.
Shepherd J, Blauw GJ, Murphy M, et al., on behalf of the PROSPER study group. Pravastatin in elderly individuals at risk of vascular disease (PROSPER): a randomised controlled trial. Lancet 2002;360:1623–1630.

Chapter 8
New Issues in the Screening and Prevention of Cardiovascular Disease

Brian V. Reamy

Aspirin Prophylaxis

The prevention of cardiovascular disease is optimized by blood pressure control, weight management, and tobacco cessation in addition to the reduction of elevated serum lipids. Even greater risk reduction can be obtained in some patients by the use of aspirin to prevent cardiovascular morbidity and mortality.

The United States Preventive Services Task Force strongly recommends that clinicians discuss the benefits of aspirin for the prevention of cardiovascular disease with their patients. It gave chemoprophylaxis with aspirin an "A" rating for patients with a greater than 3% 5-year risk of having a cardiovascular event [1]. It is important to note that the Framingham criteria computes 10-year risk, so it must be multiplied by 0.5 to get the 5-year risk.

As a general rule-of-thumb, most 40-year-old men and 50-year-old women will benefit from aspirin therapy. An important gender-specific clarification of this benefit was noted in 2006. Men have reduced cardiovascular events primarily because of a reduced incidence of myocardial infarction, whereas women benefit primarily from a reduction in the risk of stroke [2].

Patients with a 5-year cardiovascular risk of less than 3% are more likely to suffer harm than accrue benefits from aspirin therapy as a result of intracranial bleeding or gastrointestinal bleeding. Once a patient's 5-year risk surpasses 3%, they are more likely to experience benefit than harm. The benefit and harm of daily aspirin use are summarized in Table 8.1.

In contrast, the American Heart Association (AHA) recommends prophylaxis with low-dose aspirin for patients with a 10-year cardiovascular risk of 10% or greater. The AHA defines low-dose aspirin as 75 to 162 mg per day [3].

B.V. Reamy
Chair and Associate Professor, Department of Family Medicine, Uniformed Services University of the Health Sciences, Bethesda, MD
e-mail: breamy@usuhs.mil

B.V. Reamy (ed.), *Hyperlipidemia Management for Primary Care*,
DOI: 10.1007/978-0-387-76606-5_8, © Springer Science+Business Media, LLC 2008

Table 8.1 Benefits and harms of daily aspirin use

	5-year coronary heart disease risk = 1%	5-year coronary heart disease risk = 3%	5-year coronary heart disease risk = 5%
Coronary heart disease events	1–4 avoided	4–12 avoided	6–20 avoided
Hemorrhagic strokes	0–2 caused	0–2 caused	0–2 caused
Gastrointestinal bleeding events	2–4 caused	2–4 caused	2–4 caused
Overall risk:benefit ratio	Risk exceeds benefit	Benefit exceeds risk	Benefit exceeds risk

Source: Data from Recommendations of the U.S. Preventive Services Task Force: The Guide to Clinical Preventive Services, 2005. AHRQ Pub. 05-0570, pp 55–59.

Aspirin Dosage for Chemoprophylaxis

The optimal dosage of aspirin is not known. Benefits have been shown in primary and secondary prevention trials, with daily doses of 75 mg, 81 mg, 100 mg, and 325 mg every other day. Buffered or enteric-coated preparations do not seem to have clear benefits over nonbuffered aspirin formulations.

Novel Screening Tools for Risk Assessment

Although the established cardiovascular risk factors of hyperlipidemia, smoking, hypertension, family history, and diabetes accurately provide a risk assessment for more than 90% of patients, there remains a large group who could benefit from earlier preventive interventions if they could be identified by alternative screening methods. In addition, a large number of deaths from coronary disease occur suddenly and without prior symptoms [4]. Newer screening tests and methods of risk assessment could decrease this tragedy. Many serum biomarkers as well as noninvasive direct vascular imaging techniques have been studied to determine if they can identify patients earlier than traditional risk assessment.

Serum Biomarkers

Ideal serum biomarkers of risk would aid primary prevention by helping to identify individuals sooner and would aid secondary prevention by helping to guide the intensity of therapy in patients with known disease.

High Sensitivity-C-Reactive Protein (hs-CRP)

High sensitivity-C-reactive protein (hs-CRP) is the most studied and validated serum biomarker. It is an acute-phase reactant and marker of inflammation that serves as a mediator of atherosclerotic disease. Higher levels of systemic inflammation are associated with increased atherosclerosis and more unstable and vulnerable vascular plaques. It has been shown that hs-CRP is a stronger predictor of future cardiac events than low density lipoprotein (LDL). It also identifies individuals at risk in spite of low LDL levels, is of particular use in women, and adds prognostic information to the Framingham risk assessment [5].

hs-CRP can be drawn at any time of the day, and fasting is not required. It has long-term stability for risk prediction. A risk gradient exists on the basis of hs-CRP levels across all levels of traditional Framingham risk. It predicts risk independently of age, smoking, lipid levels, glucose levels, and blood pressure. The American Heart Association issued guidelines for clinicians in 2003 [6]. The AHA stated that hs-CRP should be used for additional risk assessment in those patients judged at intermediate risk by Framingham criteria. They believed that risk assessment would not change for those at high or very low risk.

Interpretation of hs-CRP is performed as follows: levels less than 1 mg/l are considered low risk; levels of 1 to 3 mg/l are intermediate risk; and levels greater than 3 mg/l are judged high risk. One caveat is that levels greater than 10 mg/l are so elevated that a clinician should search for other major inflammatory processes such as collagen vascular disease or cancer or a serious infection.

However, there are no prospective outcome trials demonstrating that reducing hs-CRP will prevent cardiovascular disease morbidity and mortality. The JUPITER trial started in 2003 with a projected conclusion in 2008; it is using rosuvastatin in a double-blind placebo-controlled trial to treat patients with elevated hs-CRP but with average LDL cholesterols. This trial will be the first to provide outcome data on the utility of lowering elevated hs-CRP with statins.

Indirectly, a subanalysis of data from the PROVE-IT trial showed that patients who had low hs-CRP levels after treatment with statins had better outcomes than those with higher hs-CRP levels, regardless of the effect on LDL level [7].

In addition to statins, anything that decreases inflammation will also lower hs-CRP, including weight loss, glucose control, blood pressure control, smoking cessation, and aerobic exercise, all of which decrease hs-CRP.

Until outcome studies are available, it seems prudent to test patients at *intermediate risk* based on Framingham assessment and to lower hs-CRP in those found to be at intermediate or high risk by hs-CRP (levels greater than 1 mg/l). hs-CRP can be lowered with therapeutic lifestyle changes or by treatment with statins.

Apolipoprotein A-1

Apolipoproteins are proteins associated with lipids that assist with their assembly, transport, and metabolism. Apolipoprotein A-1 is found on the outer layer of high density lipoprotein (HDL) and is a marker for active HDL. Many believe that it may be critical to the antioxidant and antiinflammatory properties of HDL. It also promotes cholesterol efflux from the macrophage and returns it to the liver for excretion.

Studies have shown that apolipoprotein A-1 has an independent and inverse relationship to coronary heart disease risk and is, in fact, superior to LDL as a predictor of risk. However, no clinical outcome studies have proven that increasing this biomarker will reduce clinical events.

Apolipoprotein B

Apolipoprotein B exists on the outer layer of LDL and very low density lipoprotein (VLDL) and is a marker for the total atherogenic particle concentration. Studies have shown that elevations of apolipoprotein B are directly linked to coronary risk and that it is more predictive of risk than LDL [8]. A level greater than 120 mg/dl is greater than the 75th percentile and considered high risk.

Apolipoprotein B can be computed from patients in a nonfasting state and is less expensive than a conventional lipid profile, making it a very practical test. It is a marker that is likely to become a foundation of risk assessment in the future. It has not been incorporated into the National Cholesterol Education Program (NCEP) guidelines because, similar to other novel biomarkers, there are no clinical outcome studies proving that decreasing apolipoprotein B will reduce clinical events. Additionally, there are no clear clinical "cutpoints" to help clinicians determine at which levels to provide which type and intensity of treatment.

Statins reduce levels of apolipoprotein B but, in contrast to LDL, the levels of apolipoprotein B remain predictive of risk even during treatment with statins. Elevated levels are also found with other proinflammatory states such as obesity, insulin resistance, and hypercoagulability.

Lipoprotein-a

Lipoprotein-a binds to highly atherogenic oxidized phospholipids and is a specific and independent marker for cardiovascular disease risk. It is decreased by the same factors that increase HDL: niacin, fibrates, smoking cessation, and aerobic exercise. A level greater than 39.0 mg/dl is considered the 90th percentile in Caucasian men, and 39.5 mg/dl is the 90th percentile in Caucasian women [9]. Recently, it has become clear that the 90th percentile values appear to be higher in African Americans and lower in groups of Asian ethnicity, making interpretation of lipoprotein-a measurements difficult at present.

Lipoprotein-a is a useful biomarker to assess in patients with unexplained premature coronary disease or in those who have hyperlipidemia refractory to conventional treatment with LDL-lowering agents [10]. Niacin appears to be the only pharmacologic agent capable of lowering lipoprotein-a. But, similar to other novel biomarkers, there are no clinical outcome studies that prove that lowering lipoprotein-a will reduce clinical outcomes.

Lipoprotein-Associated Phospholipase A2 (Lp-PLA2)

Lp-PLA2 is an enzyme produced mainly by macrophages and is a marker for inflammation. Similar to hs-CRP, elevated levels of Lp-PLA2 are predictive of future coronary events [11]. This association is independent from and in addition to the level of hs-CRP. It is hoped that the risk attributable to Lp-PLA2 may be additive to the risk assessment provided by hs-CRP. No clinical outcome studies are available yet.

Homocysteine

High levels of homocysteine are epidemiologically linked to future coronary events. Homocysteine is also easily decreased by folic acid supplementation. However, recent trials have dampened enthusiasm for measuring or tracking homocysteine levels as a marker for risk.

Two studies in secondary prevention suggested a harmful effect from using folate to reduce homocysteine levels. The treatment groups, despite a decrease in homocysteine levels, had increases in unstable angina and other harmful clinical effects.

B-Type Natriuretic Peptide (BNP)

BNP is a neurohormonal marker produced during times of cardiac stress, including ischemia and heart failure. As such, it is a direct marker of cardiac risk. A 2006 study showed that it was slightly superior to hs-CRP as a predictor of cardiac death or major cardiovascular events [12]. However, there are no clinical outcome trials showing that reducing BNP will reduce clinical events.

Vascular Imaging Techniques

Electron Beam Computed Tomography (EBCT)/Multislice CT Scanners

EBCT uses computed tomography (CT) to measure the amount of calcium in the coronary arteries as a surrogate for the extent of atherosclerotic vascular disease. It delivers a significant dose of radiation that can increase the risk of cancer with multiple examinations. The test is used to generate a measure termed the Calcium Score [13] (Table 8.2).

The clinical utility of EBCT remains incompletely established because the Calcium Score measures hard calcified atherosclerotic plaque better than it measures less fibrotic and more vulnerable plaque that is more likely to rupture and trigger clinical events. The vulnerable plaque that triggers most coronary events is *not* calcified or necessarily obstructive and therefore is not measured by EBCT. EBCT has not yet been able to improve upon existing techniques of disease identification or improve mortality.

Table 8.2 Interpretation of coronary calcium score

Coronary calcium score	Coronary disease likelihood
0–10	Very unlikely
11–100	Mild disease is likely
101–400	Nonobstructive disease is highly likely
Greater than 400	High likelihood of at least one obstructive lesion

The U.S. Preventive Services Task Force (USPSTF) recommends against routine screening with EBCT for the prediction of coronary events, giving it a "D" recommendation. They found that EBCT was more likely to generate significant false positives requiring additional invasive testing that is more likely to cause harm than good [1].

The American Heart Association (AHA) reviewed the available data on coronary Calcium Scores in 2007. They did not recommend the use of EBCT in patients at low risk for screening. They also did not recommend its use in patients already judged to be at high risk by traditional risk factor assessment. They stated that it may be reasonable to consider the use of a Calcium Score to further risk stratify a patient at intermediate risk [14].

Recently, the BELLES Trial used aggressive statin therapy to lower LDL cholesterol. Despite the dramatic reduction in LDL and clinical events, the coronary Calcium Score did not change among the treated patients [15,16].

Carotid Intimal Thickness (IMT)

IMT uses ultrasound to directly image the arterial wall. Many trials have established that reductions in IMT progression are correlated with reductions in coronary risk when using a variety of pharmacologic interventions to reduce risk, such as statins to reduce LDL [16]. Carotid artery intima-media thickness (IMT) measured by ultrasound predicts coronary disease-related clinical events in subjects without clinically evident disease. In contrast to the more publicized EBCT, most experts view IMT as a safer and more reliable method to measure the extent of atherosclerotic disease and the effect of therapy on disease regression or progression. A meta-analysis of IMT published in 2007 showed that IMT is a reliable marker of systemic atherosclerosis and a strong predictor of future vascular events. This reliability was limited for younger individuals compared to older patients [17].

Summary

Conventional risk factor assessment by the use of the Framingham criteria is sufficient to assess risk in more than 90% of patients. However, it misses some patients at high risk and delays the chances for earlier primary prevention. Most likely, future risk assessment will incorporate several novel biomarkers in addition to the lipid profile. Because of their low cost, availability, and the fact that the patient need not fast, tests for levels of hs-CRP, apolipoprotein B, and apolipoprotein A-1 are most likely to be incorporated into risk assessment algorithms. Clinical outcome trials are required for each of these biomarkers to identify levels that mandate treatment and to show that treatment of abnormal levels leads to a reduction in clinical events. The JUPITER trial should provide the first clinical information about hs-CRP and go a long way toward solidifying or negating its relevance as an additional biomarker for risk assessment.

References

1. Recommendations of the U.S. Preventive Services Task Force: The Guide to Clinical Preventive Services, 2005. AHRQ Pub. 05-0570, pp 55–59.
2. Berger JS, Roncaglioni MC, Avanzini F, et al. Aspirin for the primary prevention of cardiovascular events in women and men. JAMA 2006;295:306–313.
3. American Heart Association. Primary Prevention in the Adult. 2003. Available at http://www.americanheart.org/presenter.jhtml?identifier=4704. Accessed on December 18, 2006.
4. Meyerburg RJ, Interian A Jr, Mitrani RM, et al. Frequency of sudden cardiac death and profiles of risk. Am J Cardiol 1997;80:10F–19F.
5. Ridker PM. High sensitivity C-reactive protein and cardiovascular risk: rationale for screening and primary prevention. Am J Cardiol 2003;92:17 K–22 K.
6. Pearson TA, Mensah GA, Alexander RW, et al. Markers of inflammation and cardiovascular disease: a statement from the Centers for Disease Control and Prevention and the American Heart Association. Circulation 2003;107:499–511.
7. Ridker PM, Cannon CP, Morrow D, et al. C-reactive protein levels and outcomes after statin therapy. N Engl J Med 2005;352: 20-28.
8. Pischon T, Girman CJ, Sacks FM, et al. Non-high density lipoprotein cholesterol and apolipoprotein B in the prediction of coronary heart disease in men. Circulation 2005;112:3375–3383.
9. Danik JS, Rifai N, Buring JE, Ridker PM. Lipoprotein a measured with an assay independent of apolipoprotein a isoform size and risk of future cardiovascular events among initially healthy women. JAMA 2006;296:1363–1370.
10. Ariyo AA, Thach C, Tracy R. Lp(a) lipoprotein, vascular disease, and mortality in the elderly. N Engl J Med 2003;349:2108–2115.
11. Koenig W, Khuseyinova N, Lowel H, et al. Lipoprotein-associated phospholipase A2 adds to risk prediction of incident coronary events by C-reactive protein in apparently healthy middle-aged men from the general population. Circulation 2004;110:1903–1908.
12. Wang TJ, Gona P, Larson MG, et al. Multiple biomarkers for the prediction of first major cardiovascular events and death. N Engl J Med 2006;355:2631–2639.
13. Thompson GR, Partridge J. Coronary Calcification Score: the coronary risk impact factor. Lancet 2004;363:557–559.
14. ACCF/AHA Writing Committee. ACCF/AHA 2007 clinical expert consensus document on coronary artery calcium scoring by computed tomography in global cardiovascular risk assessment and in evaluation of patients with chest pain. Circulation 2007;115:402–426.
15. Raggi P, Davidson M, Callister TQ, et al. Aggressive versus moderate lipid-lowering therapy in hypercholesterolemic postmenopausal women. Circulation 2005;112:563–571.
16. Tardiff JC, Heinonen T, Orloff D, Libby P. Vascular biomarkers and surrogates in cardiovascular disease. Circulation 2006;113:2936–2942.
17. Lorenz MW, Markus HS, Bots ML, et al. Prediction of clinical cardiovascular events with carotid intima-media thickness: a systematic review and meta-analysis. Circulation 2007;115:459–467.

Suggested Key Readings

Berger JS, Roncaglioni MC, Avanzini F, et al. Aspirin for the primary prevention of cardiovascular events in women and men. JAMA 2006;295:306–313.
Pearson TA, Mensah GA, Alexander RW, et al. Markers of inflammation and cardiovascular disease: a statement from the Centers for Disease Control and Prevention and the American Heart Association. Circulation 2003;107:499–511.
Tardiff JC, Heinonen T, Orloff D, Libby P. Vascular biomarkers and surrogates in cardiovascular disease. Circulation 2006;113:2936–2942.

Chapter 9
Practical Approach to the Patient with Hyperlipidemia

Brian V. Reamy

Introduction

The National Cholesterol Education Program/Adult Treatment Panel (NCEP/ATP) guidelines reviewed in Chapter 2 provide an excellent evidence- based foundation for the management of hyperlipidemia. Using a consistent stepwise approach leads to better patient outcomes. All portions of the lipid profile are important to consider when assessing risk of cardiovascular disease, but it is prudent to first focus on optimizing low density lipoprotein (LDL). Most studies have proven the significant benefits of reducing LDL. Triglycerides (TG) and high density lipoprotein (HDL) are important, but they are secondary targets of therapy. An important exception is the patient with triglycerides greater than 500 mg/dl. In these patients, triglycerides should be reduced first to lower the risk of pancreatitis. Also, unless the LDL is directly measured, a very high triglyceride level makes the measurement and inter- pretation of LDL cholesterol difficult.

Serum Testing Frequency and Patient Follow-Up Frequency

All adults should have a baseline lipid profile, and the United States Preventive Services Task Force found strong level A evidence that men more than 35 years of age and women more than 45 years of age at risk of coronary disease should be screened and treated for abnormal lipids [1]. They found level B evidence for screening men and women more than 20 years of age for lipid disorders [1].

If lipids are normal, screening should be done every 5 years after that. If lipids are abnormal, then treatment with lifestyle changes and/or drug therapy should be started. If only lifestyle changes are instituted, lipids should be rechecked in 6 months to determine the impact of those lifestyle changes. If drug therapy is

B.V. Reamy
Chair and Associate Professor, Department of Family Medicine, Uniformed Services University of the Health Sciences, Bethesda, MD
e-mail: breamy@usuhs.mil

B.V. Reamy (ed.), *Hyperlipidemia Management for Primary Care*,
DOI: 10.1007/978-0-387-76606-5_9, © Springer Science+Business Media, LLC 2008

started, then lipids should be rechecked at 12 weeks to determine if therapy needs to be intensified. Although the peak effect of drug therapy may occur as soon as 6 weeks after initiation, many patients require 12 weeks to manifest the full effects of pharmacologic intervention. Any time lipids are checked, it is prudent to check liver function tests for any evidence of elevation.

If the 12-week check shows that lipids are now in an optimal range, then further lipid and liver function assays should be done at 6 months and 1 year. Once the values are stable, annual assays are all that is required. Any side effects should prompt an immediate investigation with liver functions and serum creatinine kinase if muscle side effects are reported by a patient.

If the 12-week check shows that an intensification of drug therapy is required, then tests should be repeated in 12 weeks. Once optimal lipid levels are gained, than repeat assays in 6 months and at 1 year are reasonable. See Fig. 9.1 for a helpful serum lipid testing algorithm.

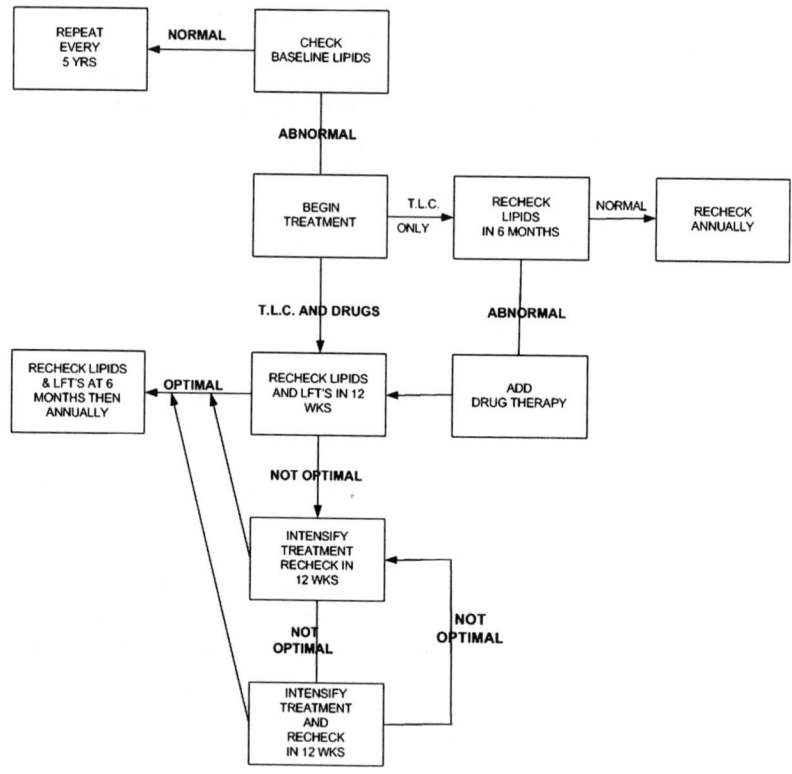

T.L.C. = THERAPEUTIC LIFESTYLE CHANGES
LFT'S = LIVER FUNCTION TESTS

Fig. 9.1 Serum lipid testing algorithm

Compliance and Motivational Tools

Long-term compliance with lipid-lowering therapy is difficult. However, the full benefits of such treatment are only realized after years of steady treatment. Several tools and strategies are helpful to assist compliance with treatment for dyslipidemia.

First, *patient education* is essential. Patients should be sent to a class that discusses the benefits of lipid-lowering therapy and allows them to ask questions. If a class is not available or in cases in which patients do not attend available classes, patients should be referred to two websites to review the information available on lipid-lowering treatments. These two sites are free, evidence based, current, and well designed for patients of diverse cultural backgrounds. The first site is the American Heart Association's page on cholesterol: http://www.americanheart.org/presenter.jhtml?identifier=1516.

This page provides excellent information and several interactive exercises as well as links to information on healthy diets, exercise, and drug treatment. The second excellent site is from the National Heart Lung and Blood Institute: http://nhlbisupport.com/chd1/how.htm.

Similar to the American Heart Association site, this page provides updated, free, evidence-based information with many interactive features. It also allows a patient to develop a cholesterol tracker and understand all the approaches to lowering serum cholesterol levels. For patients who are unable to use or access the Internet, information can be printed from these sites and made available as handouts in the office.

The second key step to help compliance is *a question-and-answer session with the physician or nurse educator* after patients have been on treatment and return for a routine follow-up visit, as discussed in the previous section. All questions should be answered, side effects should be discussed, and strategies to overcome barriers to treatment should be reviewed. Encouragement and a reemphasis on the benefits of treatment should be provided.

The third and final step to ensure compliance is a *reevaluation of risk and motivational talk*. When patients return for a follow-up serum assay, their risk should be recalculated using the Framingham risk calculator. The improvement of their risk status should be shown to the patient as a motivational tool. The physician should provide positive feedback on their successful treatment and reinforce the need for long-term compliance. A lipid tracking card, such as the one shown in Fig. 9.2, can be given to the patient to help with compliance and to remind the patient of the need for return visits. Both risk percent numbers and color codes (red = high risk, yellow = moderate risk, green = low risk) are useful to convey risk across a broad level of patient understanding. The tracking card documents improvements and helps ensure that patients know when their next visit with the doctor should take place.

Stepwise Treatment Plan

The NCEP/ATP III guidelines reviewed in Chapter 2 provide a good stepwise construct for the treatment of dyslipidemia; however, its nine steps can be lengthy and cumbersome to employ in practice [2]. The Veterans Administration and the

PATIENT NAME: _____

PATIENT DATE OF BIRTH: _____

DATE	10-Year Risk of Heart Disease	RISK	NEXT APPT.	DRUGS
1/2/2006	22%	**Highlight box in RED**	April 2006	none
4/4/2006	15%	**Highlight Box in YELLOW**	July 2006	Atorvastatin 40 mg
7/11/2006	9%	**Highlight Box in GREEN**	Jan 2007	Atorvastatin + niacin
MY GOALS	**LDL ("bad")**	**TG**	**HDL ("good")**	
	< 70	**< 150**	**> 40**	
MY VALUES				
1/2/2006	144	155	31	
4/4/2006	88	130	35	
7/11/2006	69	122	42	

Fig. 9.2 Sample lipid tracking card

Department of Defense have developed their own treatment algorithm that is outstanding in quality, but it is 25 pages long even in its briefest summary format [3]. This section provides a pragmatic modification to these guidelines and offer the author's six-step approach (Table 9.1) to the treatment of dyslipidemia. *All* patients should be instructed in healthy lifestyle changes, and LDL remains the initial target for therapy.

This six-step approach outlined in Table 9.1 is discussed in detail below.

- **Step 1:** Obtain a fasting lipid profile to include TC, TG, HDL, and LDL.
- **Step 2:** Rule out secondary causes of dyslipidemia with history and targeted lab tests as needed.
- **Step 3:** Risk Assessment. If the patient has coronary disease, diabetes, or vascular disease, he/she is at very high risk, and an LDL goal of less than 70 mg/dl, an HDL goal of more than 40 mg/dl, and a TG goal of less than 150 mg/dl are optimal. If the patient does not have coronary disease, diabetes, or vascular disease, then a Framingham risk can be calculated and the patient should be classified in one of four groups with lipid goals as shown in Table 9.2.

In patients at intermediate risk, novel serum markers of risk such as high sensitivity-C-reactive protein (hs-CRP,) apolipoprotein B, and apolipoprotein A-1 may be used to adjust the risk category up or down one level. However, as discussed in Chapter 8, outcome-based evidence of their utility is still scant.

Table 9.1 Six-step approach to hyperlipidemia

Step	Action
1	Obtain complete fasting lipid profile.
2	Rule out secondary causes of dyslipidemia.
3	Perform Framingham risk assessment. Consider novel serum markers (hs-CRP, apolipoprotein B, apolipoprotein A-1) to refine risk in those at intermediate risk.
4	Begin or intensify diet, exercise, and lifestyle modifications for all patients.
5	Begin drug therapy for patients not meeting goal LDL, HDL, and TG levels with lifestyle interventions alone. Consider statins for all patients with coronary disease or diabetes mellitus.
6	Annual reassessment of risk and continued motivation to ensure long-term compliance with treatment. Consider checking apolipoprotein B.

Table 9.2 Lipid goals according to risk category

Risk category	LDL goal	HDL goal[a]	TG goal
CHD or risk 20% or more	Less than 70 mg/dl	Greater than 40 mg/dl	Less than 150 mg/dl
Risk 10%–20%	Less than 100 mg/dl	Greater than 40 mg/dl	Less than 150 mg/dl
Two risk factors with risk less than 10%	Less than 130 mg/dl	Greater than 40 mg/dl	Less than 150 mg/dl
Zero or one risk factor	Less than 160 mg/dl	Greater than 40 mg/dl	Less than 150 mg/dl

CHD, coronary heart disease.

[a] HDL goal is greater than 50 mg/dl in premenopausal women.

- **Step 4:** Begin Therapeutic Lifestyle Changes (TLC) for *all* patients that include a healthy diet and exercise plan. (See Chapters 3, 4, and 5.) For patients with a body mass index greater than 25 kg/m [2], the diet should be developed by a dietician and promote weight loss. For all others, it should limit saturated fat, eliminate *trans* fats, and increase monounsaturated fats (tree nuts and olive oil). It should increase soluble fiber intake and encourage the consumption of a plate of food that is always brightly colored.

  At least 30 min exercise per day on most days of the week should be instituted or continued. Patients in the top two risk categories or patients older than 50 years of age should be referred for a cardiac screening test before starting an exercise program. Smoking cessation is required. For those who consume alcohol, it should be limited to one to two glasses per day, and red wine should be encouraged as the primary source of alcohol.

- **Step 5:** In cases in which the patient is at high risk, drug therapy should be instituted at the same time as TLC. In cases in which the patient is at lower risk, 6 months of TLC should be instituted first to see if goal lipid values can be reached without drug therapy. Drug selection should follow the information mentioned in Chapter 6; it can be summarized as shown in Table 9.3.

  All combination drug choices increase the risk of side effects. Hepatic enzymes should be checked any time a patient reports side effects and at 12 weeks after beginning combination therapy.

- **Step 6:** For those patients requiring treatment, an annual reassessment of risk and need to continue, reduce, or intensify therapy should be instituted. This annual reassessment should also provide an opportunity for the clinician to motivate and encourage continued compliance with the treatment plan. As noted in

Table 9.3 Drug therapy for patients and high and low lipid abnormality

Lipid abnormality[a]	First drug choice	Second drug choice	Third drug choice	Fourth drug choice
High LDL	Statin	Statin plus ezetimibe	Statin plus resin	Statin plus niacin
Low HDL	Niacin	Fibrates	Statins plus niacin or statin plus a fibrate	Niacin plus a fibrate
High TG	Fibrate	Fish oil	Niacin	Fibrate plus fish oil or niacin plus fish oil
High LDL and high TG	Statins	Statins plus niacin	Statins plus fibrates	Statins plus fish oil
Low HDL and high TG	Fibrate	Niacin	Fish oil plus a fibrate or niacin	Fish oil plus a statin combined with a fibrate or niacin
High LDL, low HDL, and high TG	Statin	Statin plus Niacin	Statin plus ezetimibe plus niacin	Statin plus ezetimibe plus a fibrate.

[a] For patients with diabetes or coronary disease, a statin agent should always be a part of their lipid-lowering regimen.

Table 9.4 Secondary causes of dyslipidemia

Cause	Effect on lipids
Hypothyroidism	Increased TG, LDL
Renal failure	Increased TG, decreased HDL
Diabetes mellitus	Increased TG, decreased HDL
HIV/AIDS	Increased TG and LDL
Nephrotic syndrome	Increased LDL
Estrogen therapy	Increased TG, decreased LDL and HDL
Diuretic therapy	Increased TG
Atypical antipsychotic therapy	Increased TG
Excessive alcohol intake	Increased TG and HDL

Chapter 8, the LDL level is a less accurate guide to risk if patients are started on statins. However, apolipoprotein B remains an accurate way to assess atherogenic particle concentration even when patients are on statin therapy.

Referral Guidelines

Most patients with dyslipidemia can be managed by primary care clinicians following the treatment guidelines suggested in this chapter. In cases of severe familial dyslipidemia or in rare cases of hyperlipidemia refractory to standard treatment, patients should be referred to endocrinologists who specialize in the treatment of lipid disorders. Before referral, compliance with therapy should be assured and possible secondary causes of hyperlipidemia should be ruled out of consideration (Table 9.4).

Partial ileal bypass was used to reduce LDL levels in patients with genetic hyperlipidemia, but it is presently only of historical interest. Patients with coronary artery disease (CAD) whose LDL remains above 200 mg/dl, or patients without CAD whose LDL remains above 300 mg/dl despite 6 months of best possible medical therapy, should be referred for LDL apheresis. This process uses a variety of techniques to filter LDL from the plasma. The procedure is similar to renal dialysis and is repeated weekly or biweekly.

References

1. US Preventive Services Task Force. The Guide to Clinical Preventive Services, 2005. AHRQ Pub. 05-0570, pp 67–70.
2. National Heart, Lung, and Blood Institute of the NIH. Third report of the National Cholesterol Education Program (NCEP) expert panel on detection, evaluation, and treatment of high blood cholesterol in adults (Adult Treatment Panel III). NIH Pub. 01-3670, May 2001.
3. VA/DoD Offices of Quality & Performance and Patient Care Services. VA/DoD Clinical Practice Guideline for the Diagnosis and Management of Dyslipidemia: Guideline Summary. 2006: http://www.oqp.med.va.gov/cpg/cpg.htm.

Chapter 10
Cases

Brian V. Reamy

Introduction

Physicians are likely to confront several common dilemmas in the management of hyperlipidemia. This chapter presents cases from actual practice to illustrate some of these dilemmas and to provide the best evidenced-based decisions grounded in the information presented in previous chapters to provide optimal care for the primary or secondary prevention of cardiovascular disease in a patient with hyperlipidemia.

CASE 1: THE WELL ELDERLY PATIENT

A healthy 82-year-old woman checked her cholesterol at a health fair and was told she needed to see her family doctor because it was high. Upon recheck with a fasting complete lipid profile, these were her test results:

TC   = 254 mg/dl
LDL = 188 mg/dl
HDL = 41 mg/dl
TG   = 125 mg/dl

Her past medical history was remarkable for some mild osteoarthritis of the knees and a 20-year history of systolic hypertension. She takes celecoxib 100 mg qd and hydrochlorthiazide 25 mg qd. She is a retired surgical nurse who lives alone in a small two-story townhouse and does all her own housekeeping. She contracted with a company to mow her small lawn. Her family history is quite remarkable. She had eight siblings. Three sisters lived to more than 100 years of age, but two sisters and three brothers had died between 50 and 80 years of age of a variety of illnesses including coronary disease and stroke.

B.V. Reamy
Chair and Associate Professor, Department of Family Medicine, Uniformed Services, University of the Health Sciences, Bethesda, MD
e-mail: breamy@usuhs.mil

B.V. Reamy (ed.), *Hyperlipidemia Management for Primary Care*,
DOI: 10.1007/978-0-387-76606-5_10, © Springer Science+Business Media, LLC 2008

Physical Examination

Her vital signs were 66 in. tall; 138 lb; pulse = 70/min; blood pressure = 158/77 mmHg.

Her examination was essentially normal for age except for some crepitus, joint line tenderness, and mild swelling of both knees.

Case Analysis

Step 1 of the NCEP/ATP guidelines is to obtain a complete and fasting lipid profile. Steps 2, 3, and 4 are to perform a risk assessment using the Framingham risk tables found at http://www.nhlbi.nih.gov. Of note, the maximum age-associated risk estimate given in these tables is for men and women up to 79 years of age; this limitation is because the Framingham data set did not follow patients greater than 80 years of age as it was much rarer that people lived that long when the study started in the 1950s. Today, living to more than 80 years in relatively good health is so common as to be routine. The Framingham risk calculator gives a 10-year risk of 27%, meaning that there is a 27% chance that she will have a cardiovascular event in the next 10 years.

Step 5 of the NCEP/ATP guidelines interprets any risk greater than 20% as very high risk and as a coronary disease equivalent, which sets her goal LDL as either less than 100 mg/dl or, optionally, less than 70 mg/dl based on recent evidence-based updates to the NCEP guidelines.

Her current LDL is 188 mg/dl; getting to goal will require a decrease from 47% to 63% in her LDL level. The TG and HDL levels are acceptable. The first step to getting to goal is *always* therapeutic lifestyle changes (NCEP Step 6). An optimal diet to include lower saturated fat and increased soluble fiber could reduce her LDL by as much as 15%. From a practical perspective, however, it can be extremely difficult to get older adults to change dietary practices that they have followed for decades. The patient's body mass index is already less than 25, so further weight loss is unlikely to significantly reduce her LDL cholesterol. It is also important to be sure that the patient is engaged in some regular physical activity.

After implementing therapeutic lifestyle changes, Step 7 is to consider adding medications to get to goal. To achieve a decrease of LDL from 47% to 63%, medications are likely to be needed. Of the medications available, only statins are likely to provide the LDL decrement required. Although most statin trials focused on adults from 45 to 65 years of age, the 2002 PROSPER Trial studied the use of statins in older patients from 70 to 82 years of age. This study provides evidence that elderly patients benefit from statin treatment to lower their LDL cholesterol with a low rate of side effects. In fact, the number needed to treat (NNT) for an 82-year-old is only 4:1, in stark contrast to a 50-year-old male, who has an NNT of approximately 35:1. This is because the prevalence of cardiovascular disease is so much greater in the elderly, making prevention more likely to provide benefits.

A retrospective study from 2002* also showed that the mortality rate for all patients more than 80 years of age taking statins was only 8.5% versus a mortality rate of 29.5% for those elderly patients not on statins.

Case Outcome

The risk assessment was discussed with the patient in terms she could understand. Although three of her sisters had lived to more than 100 years of age without treatment for high cholesterol, she was worried about her five other siblings who had died at much younger ages. She agreed that if treatment was simple and side effect free she would be happy to start it.

---

*Maycock CAA, Muhlestein JB, Horne BD et al. Statin Therapy is Associated with Reduced Mortality Across All Age Groups of Individuals with Significant Coronary Disease, Including Very Elderly Patients. J Am Coll Cardiol 2002; 40:1777-85.

Her blood pressure control was optimized by the addition of lisinopril. Given her elevated risk of cardiac disease, in accordance with USPSTF guidelines she was started on 81 mg/day aspirin. It was suggested that she stop her celecoxib and try extended-release Tylenol® for her knee pain instead, but she refused. She also refused to make any significant changes to her diet. She still did all her own housework and some seasonal gardening. It was thought that she was easily getting more than 30 min of aerobic exercise every day at an intensity appropriate for her age and her comorbidity of knee osteoarthritis. To obtain the LDL reduction desired, the potent statin atorvastatin was selected. She was started on 40 mg/day.

Twelve weeks later she was seen in clinic and reported no side effects from her medication changes. Her blood pressure was 132/74 mmHg. Her electrolytes, renal function (because of the addition of lisinopril), hepatic enzymes, and lipids were checked. Electrolytes, renal function, and liver function were normal.

Her lipids were TC = 162 mg/dl, TG = 115 mg/dl, LDL = 95 mg/dl, and HDL = 44 mg/dl. No further changes were made, and the patient was scheduled for a repeat visit in 6 months.

CASE 2: THE HEALTHY YOUNG ADULT WITH A HIGH-RISK FAMILY HISTORY

A 23-year-old medical student presented for care with a chief complaint of "I want to do something to prevent getting a heart attack." He was quite healthy with this fasting lipid profile:

TC = 243 mg/dl
TG = 120 mg/dl
LDL = 185 mg/dl
HDL = 34 mg/dl

His past medical history was remarkable for a history of moderate seasonal allergic rhinitis. He used nasal fluticasone to control his symptoms for 4 months each year. He was single and lived alone in an apartment. He did his own cooking and tried to eat what he described as a Mediterranean-style diet. He did not smoke, but he consumed two to four cups of coffee each day and a glass or two of red wine with dinner on 2 or 3 nights of the week. Of note was that he reported that he was running at least 70 miles per week at a 6-min per mile pace. He also tried to bike or swim on the weekends.

His family history was very significant. His father had died from a myocardial infarction at age 43. His two uncles had died of heart attacks as well, at ages 37 and 39 years. His paternal grandfather had died suddenly while grilling food at an outdoor barbeque at age 40. His father, by reaching age 43, was the longest-lived male relative. There was no evidence of long-QT syndrome, hypertrophic cardiomyopathy, or other congenital heart disease found in his father or uncles.

Physical Examination

His vital signs were 70 in. tall; 170 lb; pulse = 54/min; blood pressure = 126/72 mmHg.

His physical exam was remarkable for the absence of any xanthomas and for a profound brady-cardia. After rest, his pulse averaged 35 beats per minute, consistent with his history of extreme aerobic exercise.

Case Analysis

Framingham risk assessment gives him a 1% ten-year risk. Aspirin is not indicated for this low risk. According to NCEP standards, his LDL goal is less than 130 mg/dl and his HDL goal is greater than 40 mg/dl. He will require a treatment plan to increase his HDL by 18% and decrease his LDL by 30%. However, many questions and problems remain.

The NCEP guidelines are based on trials of patients more than 35 years of age, not patients this young. Because of the low prevalence of disease in this age group, it is unlikely that we will ever have prospective trials in patients this young. Starting the patient on pharmacotherapy will commit him to a lifetime of treatment with its associated risks and costs. The NNT for a patient this young is very concerning, approaching almost 250:1.

However, there is a large amount of autopsy and epidemiologic evidence from the PDAY Study, Muscatine Study, and the Bogalusa Heart Study. These studies tell us that atherosclerosis can start as early as age 2 and can progress rapidly in young adults, and this is especially true in young men who smoke or who have LDL levels greater than 160 mg/dl, as does our patient. Second, basic science studies in mammalian species confirm that atherosclerosis arrests at LDL levels less than 100 mg/dl and can reverse at levels less than 80 mg/dl.

The contribution of his devastating family history should not be overlooked. Although we do not have a quantitative way to measure this genetic risk, it is profoundly serious for this patient. What then is a reasoned approach to this patient?

Case Outcome

First, it is unreasonable to do nothing; at a minimum, intense lifestyle interventions should be undertaken. Second, the intensity of therapy must be customized to the desires of the specific patient. He was extremely knowledgeable of his genetic risk and had tried everything he could from a lifestyle perspective to lower his risk to include diet changes and extreme levels of aerobic exercise. He was very disturbed by the fact that his LDL and HDL were still abnormal despite this intervention and wanted a trial of medication. His personal desire was to reduce his LDL level to well below 100 mg/dl and to increase his HDL to greater than 40 mg/dl.

Therapeutic lifestyle changes are the key first therapeutic intervention. The patient was sent to a dietician to optimize his dietary therapy. Although his diet was judged to be quite good, several additions were made. He doubled his daily soluble fiber intake by adding oat bran, beans, and pears. He changed his red wine consumption to one or two glasses every day with dinner. He changed all his cooking oils to olive oil, eliminated two meals of beef in favor of fish, and added a handful of walnuts every day. To lessen the risk of overuse injuries, he was told to decrease his weekly mileage to 40 to 50 miles.

Simvastatin was begun at a dose of 60 mg/day with a reduction of his LDL cholesterol to 126 mg/dl and an increase of his HDL to 36 mg/dl. Although many approaches could have been taken to reduce his LDL further, a decision was made to attempt monotherapy. Therefore, the simvastatin was stopped and 80 mg/day atorvastatin was begun, with a reduction of his LDL to 109 mg/dl and an increase of his HDL to 37 mg/dl. His physician felt uncomfortable increasing his therapy any further, but the patient found another physician to add niacin at 500 mg twice per day to his regimen. Twelve weeks later his lipid profile showed LDL = 88 mg/dl and HDL = 47 mg/dl. Liver functions were normal, and the patient had no side effects so long as he took his niacin with a meal.

CASE 3: THE PATIENT WITH TYPE 2 DIABETES MELLITUS

A 55-year-old man with a 5-year history of type 2 diabetes and hypertension presented to clinic to discuss treatment of his high cholesterol. He had refused treatment in the past, but his younger brother had died of a myocardial infarction 2 weeks earlier and he decided that he should do something now. He has had several lipid profiles along with other labs in the past that average as follows:

TC   = 235 mg/dl
TG   = 185 mg/dl
HDL = 28 mg/dl
LDL = 170 mg/dl

In addition to his type 2 diabetes and hypertension, he has a history of obesity, gastroesophageal reflux, and irritable bowel syndrome. His medications were metformin, lisinopril, omeprazole, and Metamucil®. He was married and owned his own home. He had two children who were adults living away from home. He worked as a realtor and said that his job had very erratic hours and that this prevented him from eating healthy meals or exercising. His family history was significant for a history of type 2 diabetes in his father, who had died from a heart attack at age 58. His paternal grandfather had died from a myocardial infarction at age 60 and, as already noted, his brother had died 2 weeks earlier at age 52.

Physical Examination

He was an obese man who appeared mildly short of breath just moving around the examination room.

His vital signs were 69 in. tall; 268 lb; pulse = 74/min; blood pressure = 130/80 mmHg.

He had no other specific findings on physical exam and no specific signs of diabetic end-organ disease by examination.

Case Analysis

Risk assessment in this case is quite easy. By definition, diabetes is a coronary disease equivalent. He is a very high risk for disease, and he has a very deleterious lipid profile. The abnormal values in both HDL and TG in addition to LDL are quite representative of many patients with insulin resistance and type 2 diabetes mellitus.

His goals are to reduce his LDL to less than 100 mg/dl (70 mg/dl being an optional and very reasonable alternative), to reduce his TG to less than 150 mg/dl, and to increase his HDL cholesterol to greater than 40 mg/dl. In patients with diabetes, it is important to note that dyslipidemia is quite resistant to treatment unless there is optimum glucose control and an absence of other endocrinopathies such as hypothyroidism. It will be important to check a thyroid-stimulating hormone level (TSH), his glucometer records, and a hemoglobin A1C (HBA1c) before starting pharmacologic therapy for dyslipidemia.

Therapeutic lifestyle changes are essential. The patient needs to be reevaluated by a nutritional medicine consultant to select a diet for both glucose and lipid control as well as to select a diet to produce sustained weight loss to get his body mass index to less than 25 kg/m². An 1800-kcal American Diabetes Association (ADA) diet would work well for all these aims. He also needs to begin a daily exercise program. In his case, it would be important to obtain a cardiac stress test before prescribing an exercise program. His apparent lack of conditioning would mandate walking as the preferred initial form of exercise.

The British Heart Protection Study (HPS) also showed that treatment with simvastatin seemed to help diabetic patients regardless of the numerical effect on lipid values. The 2004 CARDS study showed the benefit of atorvastatin in type 2 diabetics for the primary prevention of cardiac disease regardless of the numerical effect on lipid values. It seems prudent to make a statin a first-line treatment in all patients with diabetes and add additional medications if needed. In patients with diabetes, it is also reasonable to begin a statin simultaneously with lifestyle changes.

Case Outcome

His TSH was normal, and the HBA1c was 7.8. Fasting blood glucose levels were averaging 140 mg/dl. A decision was made to add rosiglitazone to his metformin. A consulting dietician recommended a 1600-kcal diet for the weekdays and a 2000-kcal diet for the weekends, with an emphasis on five small "portable" meals per day to aid with healthy eating in the midst of an erratic work schedule. Aspirin at 81 mg/day was also started.

His exercise treadmill showed no ischemic changes but very poor exercise tolerance. He was begun on a walking program. He was asked to track his average daily number of steps for a week.

Once this number was determined, he was asked to increase his daily step count by 2,000 steps per day, a readily achievable goal. The plan was to eventually increase him to at least 10,000 steps per day on most days of the week.

Simvastatin was started at 40 mg/day. At 12 weeks, his liver enzymes, HBA1c, and lipids were rechecked. His lever functions were normal, and his HBA1c had decreased to 7.0; TC = 178 mg/dl, TG = 174 mg/dl, HDL = 31 mg/dl, and LDL = 112 mg/dl.

There were many options for the next step. Clearly, as the glucose control tightens and the diet and exercise plan take hold, his weight, fitness, and glucose values will improve without further medication. However, it is unlikely that his lipids will reach goal without further treatment. A fibrate could be added, a switch could be made to a more potent statin, or niacin could be started (knowing that although it will help lipids it may cause a temporary worsening of glucose control). In this case, a combination medication, Advicor®, was selected to help increase compliance. This combination of lovastatin and niacin was well tolerated by the patient and, after 12 weeks, led to a lipid profile of TC = 156 mg/dl, TG =150 mg/dl, LDL = 82 mg/dl, and HDL = 44 mg/dl.

CASE 4: THE PATIENT AT INTERMEDIATE RISK

A 45-year-old woman had a routine health examination and laboratory work. Her lipid profile showed:

TC = 203 mg/dl
TG = 155 mg/dl
HDL = 48 mg/dl
LDL = 124 mg/dl

Her past medical history was remarkable only for the fact that she had smoked about 1.5 packs of cigarettes per day for about 25 years (37.5 pack/year). She took a daily multivitamin. She also consumed four to six cups of coffee per day and one to two drinks of alcohol per day. She described her diet as "pretty good" and was engaged in no regular exercise. She was married with two children and lived with them, her husband, and a dog. She worked as a school nurse at the local high school. Her family history revealed a father who had a heart attack at age 60 and a mother who had a heart attack at age 64; both were smokers.

Physical Examination

She was an energetic, happy-appearing woman.
Her vital signs were 65 in. tall; 130 lb; pulse = 72/min; blood pressure =118/68 mmHg.
Other than tobacco staining of the fingers and teeth, her exam was unremarkable.

Case Analysis

Framingham risk assessment gives a 5% ten-year risk for a cardiac event, which places her in an intermediate-risk category and gives her an NCEP/ATP LDL goal of less than 130 mg/dl. So she is at goal for LDL, but a close inspection of the remainder of her lipid profile and history raises several concerns. Her family history is positive, her smoking history is very concerning, and her TG and HDL levels are both not at goal. According to the NCEP/ATP-III guidelines, her TG should be less than 150 mg/dl, and the optimum HDL for a premenopausal woman is greater than 50 mg/dl. This intermediate-risk profile is an ideal situation to use some of the novel serum biomarkers discussed in Chapter 8. The AHA recommends an hs-CRP as an ideal test for patients at intermediate risk to help raise or lower the necessity of treatment. Multiple prospective epidemiologic studies have proven that hs-CRP can predict an increased risk for cardiovascular events. It predicts risk independently of age, gender, or other risk factors. The CARE and AFCAPS/TEXCAPS studies both suggest that the benefit of statin therapy among those with normal LDL but high hs-CRP may be greater than for those with overt hyperlipidemia. It also appears to be of particular use in women.

If the hs-CRP is elevated, this would justify a more intense therapeutic intervention for primary prevention. Weight loss, smoking cessation, aerobic exercise, and statins all can lower hs-CRP.

Case Outcome

Therapeutic lifestyle changes were begun to optimize her TG and HDL and reduce her risk. She was referred to a nutritional medicine consultant who worked with her on a mutually agreeable diet that increased the amount of soluble fiber, fruits, and vegetables and reduced saturated fat. A program of walking for 30 min each day with her dog was started. The patient actually began to enjoy this daily walk as a way to "decompress" after work. She also reported that her dog was happier. Her daily intake of alcohol was changed to red wine, and a smoking cessation program was started. An hs-CRP was drawn and returned at 3.2 mg/l, equivalent to a high risk.

After 6 months, the diet and exercise program had continued, but the smoking cessation had failed despite the employment of several different methodologies and adjunctive medications. The patient had reduced her daily cigarettes to 0.5 pack per day from 1.5 packs by focusing on smoking only those cigarettes that she "truly enjoyed."

A repeat lipid profile showed that her HDL had increased to 50 mg/dl and her TG had decreased to 135 mg/dl; her hs-CRP was now in the low- to moderate-risk range at 1.4 mg/l. The patient refused further smoking cessation efforts. A plan was made to follow annual laboratory values and consider a statin if the hs-CRP increased to greater than 3.0 mg/l or if her LDL cholesterol increased to greater than 130 mg/dl.

CASE 5: THE VERY LOW GOAL LDL CHOLESTEROL

A 60-year-old man returned 3 months after a four-vessel coronary artery bypass graft (CABG) procedure. He reports that he feels "great," but that at his last visit with his cardiothoracic surgeon he was told to follow up with his family doctor to get his cholesterol in control. He was started on 20 mg/day simvastatin postoperatively. His most recent lipid profile showed:

TC = 180 mg/dl
TG = 100 mg/dl
HDL = 42 mg/dl
LDL = 118 mg/dl

In addition to coronary artery disease, his past medical history is significant for a 20-year history of hypertension, erectile dysfunction, mild osteoarthritis of his hips, and benign prostatic hypertrophy. His current medications were 325 mg aspirin per day, metoprolol 50 mg bid, simvastatin 20 mg per day, and Viagra® as needed. In addition to his four-vessel CABG, a transurethral resection of his prostate was done 2 years earlier. His family history was significant for a stroke in his father at age 68. He lived with his wife and was a retired military officer who currently taught some management classes at the local community college.

Physical Examination

His vital signs were 70 in. tall; 160 lb; pulse = 60; blood pressure = 124/76 mmHg.

His lung exam showed slightly decreased breath sounds bilaterally; his heart demonstrated a regular rate and rhythm without murmurs, rubs, or gallops. He had a well-healed central chest sternotomy scar. His extremities demonstrated no edema.

Case Analysis

Risk assessment for this patient is simple. He has coronary disease, so all interventions will be aimed at secondary prevention and maximal therapy, with an LDL goal of less than 70 mg/dl. This goal is supported by numerous trials to include the PROVE-IT Trial, which demonstrated the superiority of an LDL of 62 mg/dl over that of 95 mg/dl in secondary prevention, and the TNT and IDEAL Trials. Basic science studies also strongly suggest that, at an LDL less than 80 mg/dl, atherosclerosis can reverse.

Although his HDL and TG are at goal, his LDL needs to be decreased by another 40% in a patient already on a statin. Of note, the rule of sixes applies: doubling of a statin dose tends to only increase the LDL lowering by 6% more. So, doubling or tripling the simvastatin dose will give only 12% more LDL reduction, not the 40% needed. To get to LDL levels under 70 mg/dl, combination therapy is almost certainly needed.

As described in Chapter 6, there are five major classes of cholesterol-lowering agents, and 8 of the possible 10 class combinations have been studied and are beneficial but carry a slightly greater risk of side effects. It is important to avoid the combination of a statin with gemfibrozil, but a statin can be safely combined with fenofibrate. Many other combinations could be tried, or combination medicines such as Vytorin® or Advicor® could be prescribed. The key is to find the least complicated option that reduces LDL to less than 70 mg/dl while avoiding side effects in the patient.

Case Outcome

Therapeutic lifestyle changes were continued in line with the patient's extensive postoperative cardiac rehabilitation program. A strict vegetarian diet similar to the Ornish diet was discussed with the patient, but he believed his diet was good enough and he did not want to make such a dramatic change in his lifestyle. He was walking 5 days a week and lifting weights on 2 days of the week. Maximum strength Vytorin® was started, and his LDL decreased to 88 mg/dl. Subsequently, niacin at 500 mg twice per day was added, and the patient had a significant improvement in his lipid profile, with both a reduction in his LDL cholesterol to less than 70 mg/dl and an increase in his HDL cholesterol to 50 mg/dl.

CASE 6: CHILDREN

A 36-year-old mother brings in her two boys, aged 16 months and 6 years of age, to get their lipid profiles checked. Their 35-year-old father just underwent a five-vessel cardiac artery bypass graft procedure after suffering a heart attack. His surgeon told him that "you had better get your kids checked."

The boys' past medical history was negative. Their family history was highly significant, with multiple male relatives having suffered cardiac and vascular disease events before the age of 55 years. In addition, the mother reported that all these male relatives had abnormal cholesterol profiles. The boys lived at home with their mother, father, and grandmother. The mother and father both worked outside the home. The father was a groundskeeper at a local golf course, and the mother worked as a sales clerk at a local store. The boy's maternal grandmother lived with them and did the cooking, housekeeping, and child care until the mother returned from work each day. The mother and father both smoked a "few cigarettes every day just to relax." The mother reported, however, that since her husband's heart attack no one had been smoking.

The physical examination of both boys was age appropriate and without xanthomas.

Case Analysis

The assessment of lipid profiles in children should only be undertaken if the physician knows what they will do with the results. If not, children at high risk of premature atherosclerosis should be referred to a specialist for evaluation and treatment. It is important to realize that not all pediatric endocrinologists or pediatric cardiologists are comfortable with the treatment of pediatric hyperlipidemia.

At present, it is best to check lipid profiles only in children at high risk of premature coronary disease. It is also important that a lipid profile is not checked in a child before the age of 24 months because elevated lipids are normal and are required for normal growth and development before this age. In this case, the 16-month-old should not have his lipids checked; most likely the values can be inferred from his older sibling because the history is very suggestive of a familial combined hyperlipidemia syndrome. The 6-year-old boy's lipid profile showed:

TC   = 330 mg/dl
TG   = 210 mg/dl
HDL = 58 mg/dl
LDL = 230 mg/dl

This profile is abnormal in every respect. Recent epidemiologic surveys suggest that a 6-year-old's lipid profile should run 20 to 30 mg/dl below that of an adult. Risk assessment is difficult for this age group, but the family history and lipid profile suggest a situation in which primary prevention could help slow the onset of clinical cardiovascular disease.

As discussed in the case of the young adult earlier in this chapter, the PDAY, Muscatine, and Bogalusa Heart Studies all suggest that atherosclerosis can start as early as age 2 and can progress very rapidly in the presence of hypertension, hyperlipidemia, or smoking. Given this child's lipid profile and family history, it seems that some intervention for primary prevention of atherosclerotic heart disease is warranted.

Therapeutic lifestyle changes are safe and effective for all age groups. It is important that in children the changes are focused on unhealthy parental lifestyles as well, because the parents or adult caregivers are usually the primary providers of food and have a large impact on the risk of smoking and physical inactivity in their children.

The only medications that are FDA approved for use in children are resins. However, compliance with resins in children is extremely problematic. The gritty texture, abdominal bloating, and flatulence are all problematic. Most believe that statins are safe after puberty. As discussed in Chapter 6, there is a growing level of experience with statins in children as young as age 8 years. In limited trials over 2 years, several statins appear safe and effective.

Case Outcome

The mother was very concerned about her sons and very motivated to make significant lifestyle changes. First, the mother and father were referred to a formal smoking cessation program. Second, the mother and grandmother (the latter was the primary food preparer) were referred to a dietician for discussion of a healthier diet for all members of the family that lowers amounts of saturated fat and simple sugars and increases amounts of fruits and vegetables.

Third, a physical activity diary was performed. Based on this diary, the television watching and computer-gaming times of the children were limited to 2 h per day maximum. The 6-year-old was given a new bicycle. Daily walks with the family dog were started. A program of annual checks of the children's blood pressure, body mass index, and physical activity was started.

Although medications would be required to reduce the lipids to healthier levels, it was thought to be too early to safely begin medications. It was decided that at age 8 the children would be referred to a local specialist for consideration of pharmacologic treatment with a statin. It is hoped that even more trial information of the safety or risks of the use of statins would be available by then. The parents were told that certainly after puberty it would be safe to begin treatment with statins in the two boys. Of note: If the children had been high-risk girls, pregnancy prevention would be another important issue to consider if a statin prescription were used.

CASE 7: HIGH TRIGLYCERIDES, LOW HDL, AND METABOLIC SYNDROME

A 43-year-old man presented to his physician for a routine checkup. His father had died a few months earlier from a sudden cardiac death at age 62. His past medical history was significant for a history of gastroesophageal reflux and hypertension for 3 years. He currently used lisinopril 20 mg/day and lansoprazole every day. He was married and lived with his wife and one child in a townhouse. He was an attorney for the U.S. Government. He did not smoke and drank a martini 3 or 4 nights of the week. He said he did not have time for exercise. In addition to his father's death at age 62, his family history was significant for a paternal uncle who had undergone a coronary procedure at age 53 for a blocked coronary artery. The patient was not sure what type of procedure it was and did not have any other history about his uncle. His labs showed the following:

TC = 198 mg/dl
TG = 240 mg/dl
LDL = 129 mg/dl
HDL = 21 mg/dl

Fasting glucose = 105 mg/dl (remainder of chemistry profile was normal)

Physical Examination

His vital signs were 71 in. tall; 210 lb; waist circumference = 36 in.; pulse = 74/min; blood pressure = 138/78 mmHg.

The rest of his examination was nonfocal.

Case Analysis

The patient's 10-year risk of an event is 3% based on the Framingham criteria, and he has two risk factors. Based on this risk, his LDL goal is less than 130 mg/dl: the patient is therefore at goal. However, Step 8 of the NCEP/ATP III guidelines pushes the clinician to also review the HDL and TG levels and consider if metabolic syndrome is present (Table 10.1). Based on these criteria, the patient has three of the five criteria of metabolic syndrome (TG more than 150 mg/dl, BP greater than 130 mmHg, HDL less than 40 mg/dl), which is diagnostic for metabolic syndrome.

Table 10.1 National Cholesterol Education Program (NCEP)/Adult Treatment Panel (ATP) III criteria for metabolic syndrome (any three of five risk factors)

Risk factor	Criteria
Waist circumference	
Men	More than 40 in.
Women	More than 35 in.
Triglycerides	150 mg/dl or more
HDL	
Men	Less than 40 mg/dl>
Women	Less than 50 mg/dl
Blood pressure	130/85 mmHg or higher
Fasting glucose	110 mg/dl or higher

Source: Data from the NCEP/ATP-III guidelines. NIH publication 02-3305, May 2001.

The *keys* to the treatment of metabolic syndrome are to reduce body weight to a body mass index less than $25 \, kg/m^2$ and to increase physical activity. Both these interventions help to reduce insulin resistance, which is the key physiological disturbance of metabolic syndrome.

If, despite weight loss and increased physical activity, metabolic syndrome risk factors persist, it is important to treat hypertension, to consider aspirin therapy, and to treat the increased TG and reduced HDL with drugs. It is important to note that, if the TG is greater than 500 mg/dl, this becomes the first task in treatment, because patients with TG greater than 500 mg/dl can have spontaneous episodes of pancreatitis.

The 1999 VA-HIT Study provides some of the evidence that supports the treatment of patients with normal LDL but abnormal HDL and triglycerides. As noted in Chapter 1, this study used gemfibrozil as the therapeutic intervention and produced a significant reduction in cardiovascular events in just 5 years.

As noted in Chapter 6, the key agents for reducing triglycerides are fibrates, niacin, and fish oil. Although there are no ideal agents to increase HDL, the most potent agent available is niacin. Fibrates also increase HDL. Statins can increase HDL up to 5%. Newer pharmacologic agents are needed to help increase HDL with fewer side effects.

Additionally, future years will bring further research on the benefits of preventive treatment to forestall the onset of type 2 diabetes in patients with metabolic syndrome. Metformin and the thiazolidinedione medications have been shown to delay the onset of diabetes in other patients at risk as a consequence of family history or a personal history of gestational diabetes. All these agents activate PPAR receptors in the cell, which are crucial for mediating insulin sensitivity.

Case Outcome

The patient decided to join a Weight Watchers® group that had lunchtime meetings near his office. After a normal screening exercise treadmill, he also started on a walking program designed to increase his daily activity to at least 10,000 steps. As part of this effort, he was encouraged to make three simple interventions that can add up to 2,000 steps per day for most patients. He always chose the parking space furthest from the store or office he was driving to; he always would take the stairs up or down for any trips less than or equal to three flights; he would walk around his office to speak to colleagues in person versus calling them on the telephone.

His antihypertensive therapy was augmented by the addition of a low-dose diuretic that reduced his blood pressure to a mean of 124/74 mmHg. Finally, he was started on fenofibrate at a dose of 148 mg/day. Twelve weeks later, his TC = 196 mg/dl, his LDL =133 mg/dl, his TG = 185 mg/dl, and his HDL increased minimally to 26 mg/dl. The minimal changes of his lipids despite all these therapeutic interventions are very characteristic of patients with the metabolic syndrome. The slight increase in LDL is also commonly seen in treatment with fibrates.

After discussion with the patient, it was decided to continue all the lifestyle interventions, continue the fenofibrate, and to add two other agents to his regimen. Omacor® was added to reduce his triglycerides, and niacin 500 mg twice per day was added to help increase his HDL further.

Twelve weeks later, the patient's weight had decreased, his blood pressure remained in control, and his lipid profile was TC = 186 mg/dl, LDL = 128 mg/dl, TG = 100 mg/dl, and HDL = 38 mg/dl. Compliance with his fairly intense treatment regimen over the long term was seen as the biggest challenge. He was also told that once he turned age 45 his 5-year risk for a cardiovascular event would be greater than 5%, which would require 81 mg/day aspirin as a preventive intervention.

CASE 8: HIGH LDL, BUT CANNOT USE STATINS

A 54-year-old woman with recently diagnosed type 2 diabetes presented to her physician for a routine checkup. Her past medical history was remarkable for chronic dysthymia punctuated by episodes of major depression, obesity, hypertension, and a 40-pack per year smoking history. Her medications were fluoxetine, glipizide, metformin, fosinopril, and hydrochlorthiazide. Her family history was significant for multiple relatives with type 2 diabetes and several women who had strokes before the age of 65. Her labs showed a hemoglobin A1c of 6.8 and normal chemistries with a fasting glucose of 110 mg/dl. Her lipid panel was as follows:

TC   = 230 mg/dl
TG   = 155 mg/dl
HDL = 36 mg/dl
LDL = 163 mg/dl

Physical Examination

Her vital signs were 65 in. tall; 238 lb; pulse = 80; blood pressure = 126/72 mmHg.

She was a sad-appearing, obese woman in no distress. Her examination revealed no focal abnormalities or clinical evidence of neuropathy.

Case Analysis

This patient is at very high risk because of her diabetes. Her smoking history, family history, hypertension, obesity, and abnormal lipids add even greater risk. Her goal LDL is at a minimum of less than 100 mg/dl, but recent trials would support lowering the LDL to less than 70 mg/dl in this very high risk patient.

It will be critical to reduce her weight and stop her smoking as a foundation to any pharmacologic intervention that is undertaken. It is probable that dual therapy may be required to reduce her LDL by 60% and increase her HDL by almost 40% to get it to be greater than 50 mg/dl. Daily aspirin should also be started to reduce her risk of stroke.

In some patients, side effects from lipid-lowering drugs can be quite problematic and require some creative problem solving. Atypical combinations are often required that, although safe, may have little or no clinical outcome evidence to support their use. Lifestyle interventions are even more important in these situations, including more radical interventions such as the vegan Ornish diet program in motivated patients.

Case Outcome

The patient was prescribed a 1600-kcal ADA diet for both glucose control and weight reduction. A walking program was started with a goal of increasing her walking to a point that she was walking for at least 30 min per day on at least 5 days of the week. Her physician noted that her chronic dysthymia seemed to improve as her walking became more regular and enjoyable for her.

Simultaneous with the lifestyle interventions, the patient was started on 81 mg/day aspirin and 40 mg/day simvastatin. However, she reported severe calf muscle cramps and refused to take it. Given the alternative pathway of metabolism for pravastatin, it was chosen as an alternative. Again, the patient complained of muscle aches. Statin side effects are often agent specific and not class specific, so the patient was switched to atorvastatin. However, she also had muscle aches on atorvastatin and refused to take it or any other statin medications.

The physician decided to use niacin and slowly titrate the dose to a level that controlled her dyslipidemia. The patient complained of flushing, stomach upset, and a worsening of her moods and told her physician that "you must be crazy if you think anyone can take that medicine."

At this point the patient decided to try some "natural" remedies for her dyslipidemia. She was cautioned by her physician that red fungus rice or went yeast sold in many health food stores for cholesterol lowering are in fact a natural source of statins. She chose to start on garlic and guggulipid with no significant change in her LDL level.

At this point, 1 year later she returned to her physician very frustrated. Her lipid levels were repeated and showed the benefits of her diet and exercise program with an LDL that had decreased to 144 mg/dl and an HDL that had increased to 41 mg/dl. After discussing options, ezetimibe was prescribed at 10 mg each morning along with colsevelam each evening with dinner. She was encouraged to increase the soluble fiber content of her diet by consuming at least four soluble fiber-rich foods each day. The patient had no side effects with this regimen. Her LDL decreased to 110 mg/dl and her HDL stayed at 41 mg/dl. Although not ideal, her program of lifestyle changes and drug treatment had decreased her risk substantially.

Chapter 11
Future Directions

Brian V. Reamy

Introduction

The past decades have seen evidence accumulate in favor of ever lower LDL cholesterol goals. Some worry that there is a point at which the harm of a low LDL may overtake the benefits. Additionally, newer agents are needed to help achieve these low levels of LDL and to help raise HDL. This chapter reviews some of the trends and future directions in the management of hyperlipidemia.

How Low Do You Go?

The Heart Protection Study showed that, regardless of the effect on lipid levels, statin therapy has benefits in all patients with known disease and in those patients at high risk who do not as yet have clinical manifestations of atherosclerotic vascular disease [1]. Other studies such as the PROSPER Trial also suggested the benefits of statin therapy in primary and secondary prevention regardless of the effect on lipid levels. Several investigators began to suggest that we should abandon the concept of titrating the intensity of our treatment to achieve a specific LDL level and treat patients with a fixed dose of statins.

The PROVE-IT, IDEAL, ASCOT, and TNT Trials provided opposing evidence. They showed that lower is indeed better, driving the suggested LDL goal for patients at very high risk of disease to less than 70 mg/dl [2–5]. A subsequent meta analysis of trials comparing high dose statin therapy to standard dose statin therapy also showed that intensive lowering of LDL provides a significant benefit over standard dose therapy for preventing nonfatal cardiovascular events [6]. Trials have shown a

B.V. Reamy
Chair and Associate Professor, Department of Family Medicine, Uniformed Services University of the Health Sciences, Bethesda, MD
e-mail: breamy@usuhs.mil

B.V. Reamy (ed.), *Hyperlipidemia Management for Primary Care*,
DOI: 10.1007/978-0-387-76606-5_11, © Springer Science+Business Media, LLC 2008

direct and linear correlation between lowering of LDL and the reduction of cardio-vascular events.

However, concerns remain. Intense LDL-lowering therapy often requires multiple drugs, which raises costs and the chances for serious side effects in patients. It seems clear that a decision to pursue intense LDL lowering must be coupled with patient education, good compliance, and close follow-up for any potential side effects. If side effects are caught early, they are almost always reversible and transient. It is also critical to reinforce the need for therapeutic lifestyle changes as the bedrock of intense LDL lowering. Although patients can sometimes achieve modest LDL reductions without lifestyle changes, it is very difficult to achieve LDL lowering to less than 70 mg/dl without close attention to a healthy diet, smoking cessation, and daily exercise.

At present, there has been no LDL level at which harm has been shown to outweigh benefits. But, from a practical perspective, unless new types of medications are developed, it will be difficult to push LDL levels lower in most patients. It is also essential to develop new medications to help treat the secondary targets of raising HDL and lowering TG levels.

New Drugs

Chapter 6 discussed some of the drugs of the future. Ideal agents will be potent enough to reduce LDL to less than 70 mg/dl without a need for combination therapy. New classes beyond statins may be required. Recently, a small trial demonstrated the ability of a microsomal triglyceride transfer protein inhibitor to dramatically decrease LDL levels in patients with severe familial hypercholesterolemia [7].

Additionally, agents that safely increase *functional* HDL levels are required. It has become clear that serum HDL levels are not a perfect marker for the antiatherosclerotic potential of HDL in many patients. Although the cholesterol ester transferase protein (CETP) inhibitor torceptrapib was able to dramatically increase HDL, it led to overall harm, probably because the type of HDL produced was not antiatherosclerotic, functional HDL. Other drugs that may help increase HDL include macrophage-ATP-binding cassette transporter A1 (ABCA1) promoters and recombinant apo-A1 Milano. Apo-A1 Milano mimics highly functional HDL and causes dramatic plaque regression with intravenous infusion.

It is known that perioxisome proliferators activated receptor (PPAR)-α receptors turn on HDL. Agents that activate PPAR-α receptors to a greater degree than fibrates or niacin are clearly needed. PPAR activation is also a way to decrease insulin resistance and mediate lower blood sugars. It is also probable that PPAR activation will be a more effective way to treat the multimodal morbidity of metabolic syndrome by helping to reduce glucose, lipids, and body weight.

Integrative Treatment

The best drugs in the world will not work if patients forget to take them or do not comply with long-term treatment. Even in the best of circumstances, only 49%

of patients continue with long-term lipid-lowering therapy. Great inroads into the prevention of cardiovascular disease can be produced by developing an integrated healthcare delivery system that provides the patient with a culturally appropriate, multimodal treatment plan.

This plan would involve diet, exercise, and smoking cessation information delivered in a way that is understood by the patient and follows some of the information provided in Chapters 3, 4, and 5. In cases in which a clinician does not have the time or expertise to provide lifestyle information, it is critical that nutritional medicine consultants, sports medicine physicians, and behavioral health providers be integrated into a seamless plan of referral and communication with the patient and primary physician. When patients sense that all members of the healthcare team are focused on a similar goal, compliance with treatment increases dramatically.

Handouts, websites, and individual cards showing treatment results, medications, and time for future appointments should be given to patients, as described in Chapter 9. All these interventions can help to motivate long-term behavior change.

Integrative treatment also requires physicians to leave behind a "silo" model of treating disease. Commonly, a single patient develops individual conditions spread out over many years. Each condition is seen as requiring an individual treatment plan. Thus, a patient will be given a plan for his hypertension, an individual treatment plan for his hyperlipidemia, an individual treatment plan for his obesity, and individualized treatment plans for other comorbidities. This multiplicity of plans overwhelms physicians as well as patients, who have trouble keeping track of multiple plans and treatments.

It is important to change this mindset into a more integrative frame of reference. The clinical question *should not be*: What is the best medication for treating hypertension or hyperlipidemia? The question *should be*: What is the best treatment plan to reduce the risk of cardiovascular disease? Physical inactivity, obesity, glucose intolerance, hypertension, hyperlipidemia, and tobacco abuse are *all* risk factors and manifestations of the same problem—cardiovascular disease. Cardiovascular disease remains the number one killer of patients because we approach each of these risk factors from a "silo" versus an integrative perspective. In the end, the goal is not to lower blood pressure to less than 130/80 mHg or LDL to less than 70 mg/dl; the goal is to prevent heart attack and stroke.

What would an ideal integrative plan institute? It would mean that the patient who is diagnosed with hypertension at age 31, does not smoke, is not obese, has a normal glucose level, and has an LDL less than 130 mg/dl is not just placed on an antihypertensive medication and sent on his/her way with annual follow-up. Instead, he/she would be evaluated by a team designed to help reduce overall cardiovascular risk. Dramatic dietary changes are made just as if he/she had hyperlipidemia. An exercise plan is developed for him/her to increase HDL, lower TG, and lower fasting glucose just as if he/she were inactive and diabetic. The hazards of smoking are restated. Early, multimodal intervention is the only way to combat the "silo" approach to cardiovascular disease, which clearly does not work.

In effect, instead of an approach in which each manifestation of cardiovascular risk is treated as it becomes clinically apparent, the integrative approach would provide a full prescription or an R *for cardiovascular disease prevention*. This R would include dietary advice for healthy eating, with caloric restriction advice to get the BMI below 25 kg/m² (if needed), an exercise prescription, smoking cessation information (if needed), and, last, any medications required.

Many would take this shattering of "silos" even further and believe that the onset of any of the major cardiovascular risk factors should prompt aggressive intervention for all risks with medications. The "polypill" concept is the most dramatic manifestation of this idea [8]. In this model of integrated treatment, *all* patients diagnosed with hypertension *or* hyperlipidemia *or* diabetes would be placed on a single "polypill" containing statins, an angiotensin-converting enzyme inhibitor, aspirin, and metformin or a thiazolidinedione to forestall or prevent cardiovascular disease. Although clinical outcome evidence does not yet exist to fully support this approach, there are many intriguing studies suggesting that this pharmacologic "silo-busting" is a coming wave of treatment in the future.

Finally, patients need to learn to take charge of their own therapy and ultimately become more knowledgeable of their individual risk profile and treatment plan than any member of their care team. They should continue to improve their lifestyle through exercise and smart dietary choices and share their knowledge with family and friends. In the end, patients should understand that the "front-line" worker in the control of their cardiac risk is *not* their family doctor: It is they themselves!

References

1. Heart Protection Study Collaborative Group. MRC/BHF Heart Protection Study of Cholesterol Lowering in 20,536 high-risk individuals: a randomized placebo controlled trial. Lancet 2002;360:7–22.
2. Pedersen TR, Faergeman O, Kastelein JJP, et al. High-dose atorvastatin vs. usual-dose simvastatin for secondary prevention after myocardial infarction. IDEAL study: a randomized controlled trial. JAMA 2005;294:2437–2445.
3. Sever PS, Dahlof B, Poulter NR, et al. Prevention of coronary and stroke events with atorvastatin in hypertensive patients who have average or lower than average cholesterol concentrations in the Anglo-Scandinavian Cardiac Outcomes Trial–Lipid Lowering Arm (ASCOT-LLA). Lancet 2003;361:1149–1158.
4. LaRosa JC, Grundy SM, Waters DD, et al. Intensive lipid lowering with atorvastatin in patients with stable coronary disease. N Engl J Med 2005;352:1425–1435.
5. Cannon CP, Braunwald E, McCabe CH, et al. Intensive versus moderate lipid lowering with statins after acute coronary syndromes. N Engl J Med 2004;350:1495–1504.
6. Cannon CP, Steinberg BA, Murphy SA, et al. Meta-analysis of cardiovascular outcomes trials comparing intensive versus moderate statin therapy. J Am Coll Cardiol 2006;48:438–445.
7. Cuchel M, Bloedon LT, Szapary PO, et al. Inhibition of microsomal triglyceride transfer protein in familial hypercholesterolemia. N Engl J Med 2007;356:148–156.
8. Wald NJ, Law MR. A strategy to reduce cardiovascular disease by more than 80%. BMJ 2003;326:1419–1423.

Index

Italicized Page numbers refer to tables

A

ABCA1, *see* Adenosine triphosphate-binding
    cassette protein A1 (ABCA1)
Abdominal adiposity, 39
ACSM's Guidelines for Exercise Testing and
    Prescription, 120
Acute *vs.* chronic effect of exercise, 117
Adenosine triphosphate-binding cassette
    protein A1 (ABCA1), 157, 216
Adherence LDL-lowering, interventions to
    improve, *35*
Adults below 35 years, hyperlipidemia
    prevention, 172–173
Adult Treatment Panel III (ATP III), 15, 21–37,
    73, 172, 178, 179, 195
  new features, *19*
  normal lipid values, *19*
Agents, effects/dosage/usage (drug treatment)
  absorption inhibitors, 136
  combination agents, 141–142
    more than two, 143–144
  fibrate, 138
  fibrates plus niacin, 143–144
  fish oil, 140–141
  niacin, 137–138
  resins/bile acid sequestrants, 134–136
  statins, 138–140
  used in combination
    fibrates plus niacin, 143–144
    resins plus fibrates, 143
    resins plus niacin, 143
    statin combinations, 143
AHA, *see* American Heart Association (AHA)
ALE, *see* Artichoke leaf extract (ALE)
Allium sativum, see Garlic, studies on
American Academy of Family Physicians
    (AAFP), 126

American Heart Association (AHA), 51, 174,
    185, 190
The American Heart Association and the
    American College of Cardiology
    (AHA/ACC), guidelines for
    prevention, 11
American heart association diet and lifestyle
    recommendations revision 2006, 58
  goals, 59–60
  specific dietary recommendations, 60–62
Americans In Motion (AIM), 126
  patient counseling, implementation of AIM
    program, 126–127
  program summary, *127*
Apolipoprotein A-1, 188
  See also Tools, risk assessment
Apolipoprotein B, 188
  See also Tools, risk assessment
Artichoke, 100
  See also Therapeutic foods
Artichoke leaf extract (ALE), 100
ASCVD, *see* Atherosclerotic Cardiovascular
    Disease (ASCVD)
Aspirin prophylaxis, 185–186
Aspirin use (daily), benefits and harms, *186*
ASPVD, *see* Atherosclerotic Peripheral
    Disease (ASPVD)
Atherosclerosis, age of start
  Bogalusa Heart Study, 2
  Muscatine Study, 2
  PDAY, 2
Atherosclerotic cardiovascular disease
    (ASCVD), 113, 172, 179–180
Atherosclerotic Peripheral Disease (ASPVD),
    179, 180
Atkins, Dr. Robert, 40

Printed in the United States